"Occupational therapy in Canada stands at a pivotal juncture, where the importance of effective collaboration between occupational therapists (OTs) and occupational therapist assistants (OTAs) cannot be overstated. Heather Gillespie, whose extensive career and contributions have significantly shaped the discourse on OT-OTA collaboration, is a prominent figure in this endeavor. Heather has consistently championed the integration of OTAs into the professional practice landscape.

The significance of this topic is underscored by the findings of my doctoral work, which highlighted a critical need for resources and interventions that support OT-OTA intraprofessional collaboration. Throughout my work, I frequently heard the importance of OT-OTA intraprofessional collaboration emphasized, not only as a means to ensure access to necessary occupational therapy services, but also for its positive impact on client and organizational outcomes, and for the future of occupational therapy. As healthcare delivery evolves, this book marks the first resource in Canada that provides strategies to enhance intraprofessional collaboration in occupational therapy, promoting a more inclusive and effective practice for the benefit of all Canadians."

Dr. Teresa R. Avvampato, MSc(OT), DSc,
Professor and Researcher,
OTA & PTA Program, Faculty of Health Sciences (HS),
Durham College,
Oshawa, Ontario

T0334174

Optimal Collaboration for the Occupational Therapist and Occupational Therapist Assistant

This book acts as a guide for occupational therapists to develop and continually evaluate trusting working relationships with occupational therapist assistants (OTAs), resulting in more effective occupational therapy service delivery to clients. To combat the misunderstandings between occupational therapists and OTAs, this book provides theoretical knowledge, practical learning, and case study examples to guide and develop positive working relationships between occupational therapists and OTAs. The importance of developing this trusting intraprofessional relationship is discussed in detail, and recommended approaches are reviewed. Described methodologies can be utilized to determine appropriate involvement of OTAs in specific client treatments, allowing for a consistent and effective synergy within occupational therapy. This book is an ideal read for occupational therapist students and occupational therapists currently working in a clinical practice setting, as well as for rehabilitation managers and employers. It is also a beneficial resource for OTA students and OTAs working within the profession.

Heather Gillespie, B.O.T., has been an occupational therapist in Canada since 1977 and has collaborated with OTAs throughout her career. She currently teaches OTA students online through Medicine Hat College in Alberta.

Optimal Collaboration for the Occupational Therapist and Occupational Therapist Assistant

Heather Gillespie

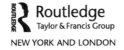
Routledge
Taylor & Francis Group

NEW YORK AND LONDON

Designed cover image: ©Getty Images

First published 2025
by Routledge
605 Third Avenue, New York, NY 10158

and by Routledge
4 Park Square, Milton Park, Abingdon, Oxon, OX14 4RN

Routledge is an imprint of the Taylor & Francis Group, an informa business

ISBN: 978-1-032-81157-4 (hbk)
ISBN: 978-1-032-80189-6 (pbk)
ISBN: 978-1-003-49839-1 (ebk)

DOI: 10.4324/9781003498391

Typeset in Palatino
by SPi Technologies India Pvt Ltd (Straive)

Access the Support Material: www.routledge.com/9781032811574

Contents

Preface

Reflecting over her career as an occupational therapist in Canada, the author realizes that improving individuals' occupational participation to promote a sense of well-being would have been significantly more challenging without the valuable work of occupational therapist assistants (OTAs), or support personnel as they were previously named. OTAs' contributions to the therapeutic process are invaluable and result in more timely and effective healthcare delivery. The author has been fortunate to collaborate with these colleagues as a clinician, fieldwork supervisor, educator, manager, and mentor in various environments and geographical locations. Throughout her professional journey, she has expanded her skills and knowledge of specific interventions by being receptive to the previous experiences and new ideas of these co-workers, which in turn can only benefit those within healthcare.

Partnering with occupational therapist assistants (OTAs) in the provision of optimal client care has developed into a professional passion for the author, from which the idea of developing this book was born. Forming a collaborative relationship leads to the occupational therapist and the OTA combining their skills and knowledge to explore the meaning and purpose of occupations (CAOT, 2024, p. 2). This book will discuss the knowledge and skills required for this relationship to be successful and to ensure the collaboration continues to evolve within the occupational therapy profession.

The author was unaware of the profession of occupational therapy until she was hired as a secretary within a rehabilitation centre during the summer before her grade 12 high school year. The position was within the occupational therapy department and her role was to type the therapists' reports and treatment plans. She also had the opportunity to observe therapists providing a variety of treatments to their patients. This job sparked the author's interest in becoming an occupational therapist as she could be creative and assist people who were experiencing challenges in their daily lives. Following investigation of the educational requirements needed, she applied to the local university. She was fortunate to be accepted into the occupational therapist diploma program following grade 12 in 1974 and has enjoyed this profession ever since.

Beginning her career as an occupational therapist in 1977 in Regina, Saskatchewan, the author was able to experience the on-the-job-training model of OTAs firsthand. The rehabilitation aides, as they were titled in her initial clinical work setting at a rehabilitation centre, had been working in their roles in occupational therapy for many years; this led to their "training" the therapists in what they did, and guiding the author as to how they should be supervised when they were treating her patients. This subject was minimally addressed in university education, and although she did experience support personnel assisting with occupational therapy service delivery during fieldwork placements, there remained confusion as to their role and the therapist's responsibilities in their supervision. The mentoring and guidance from occupational therapist colleagues regarding the process for assignment of tasks and supervising OTAs was extremely beneficial as the author began her career. This soon resulted in an increase in her competence and confidence in building this intraprofessional collaboration.

Five years into her career, the author relocated to an acute care hospital that had not recently employed an occupational therapist. She was "assigned" an assistant who had worked under the supervision of physiotherapists but did not have experience working alongside occupational therapists. This was her opportunity to "train" the assistant on-the-job as deemed appropriate. Over time, a trusting and effective professional collaboration was developed which has lasted to the present day. They were able to provide competent, ethical occupational therapy as an intraprofessional team with a clear understanding of each other's roles.

It was during her next career move to another acute care setting that the formal education program for occupational therapist assistants and physiotherapist assistants (OTA & PTA) was initiated in the province. The author had again successfully trained an OTA on-the-job and was concerned about this being taken away from her, as assistants would now receive a formal college education. Her view was that she would educate assistants in what she believed they needed to know and that a formal education program was not necessary. She also felt somewhat threatened that the graduates may know more than she did, or at least be more current in their knowledge as it was approximately 18 years since she had graduated as an occupational therapist. When asked to offer a fieldwork placement for the first student cohort, the author declined, stating honestly that she was not comfortable with the ten-month formal education program. This response was accepted, but the head of the education program strongly encouraged the author to enter into a dialogue with the students who would be receiving fieldwork experiences from physiotherapist colleagues in order that she become more informed about the education program. She followed up on this and came to realize these students did have critical knowledge and skills – for example, they knew the difference between occupational therapy and physiotherapy (not common knowledge at that time for many healthcare professionals), and they were aware of various physical and mental health conditions throughout the lifespan in addition to appropriate treatment options for specific conditions. This discovery changed her thinking, and she did offer an OTA fieldwork placement the following year – and was extremely pleased with the student's performance! A few years later, the author was offered the opportunity to manage the same OTA & PTA education program, as well as to instruct the OTA courses. This offer was accepted and, as a result, further increased her understanding of the OTA role and the foundational knowledge they brought to occupational therapy. She also learned the benefits of their dual training in both occupational therapy and physiotherapy; a single OTA/PTA could therefore help clients who required treatments from both disciplines. The author believes that the turning point in her career was when she realized the critical contributions made by formally educated

OTA colleagues in assisting clients to reach their occupational participation goals.

As her own occupational therapist career continued to develop, the author began volunteering with the provincial occupational therapy association, including holding the position of President. Following this, she represented Saskatchewan as a Board Director within the Canadian Association of Occupational Therapists and has continued to be involved with CAOT on various committees and task groups, many related to increasing the involvement of OTAs within the profession.

Following a provincial relocation in 2001 to British Columbia, she was made aware that the understanding of, and confidence in, the OTA role varies within different jurisdictions. In some areas there is a greater knowledge but in other areas the inclusion of OTAs in occupational therapy service delivery is poorly understood and supported. She was fortunate to be given the opportunity to resume teaching OTAs through online delivery within the OTA/PTA Program at Medicine Hat College in Medicine Hat, Alberta in 2009 and currently continues in this instructor role. The online delivery format provides access to those residing in various locations across the country to pursue their career as an OTA/PTA from the environment where they reside, and the author continues to learn about the successes and challenges for OTAs within various jurisdictions. This experience encouraged her to create the goal of further advocating for the OTA role within this great profession across the country.

The idea of developing this book therefore came to fruition to assist all those involved in the profession of occupational therapy, including occupational therapists, occupational therapist educators, student occupational therapists, OTAs, OTA students, OTA educators, practice leaders, managers, and employers in the understanding of the OTA knowledge and skill base, critical thinking abilities, and potential roles in occupational therapy service delivery. In addition, it is imperative that all team members and those in management positions recognize, understand, and are supportive of the responsibilities and limitations of OTAs within each work environment. Furthermore, the provincial and territorial occupational therapy associations need to understand the role of OTAs by providing appropriate resources and guidance for their members. It is also important for occupational therapist regulatory organizations to comprehend the OTA role, and ensure the public is protected through the safe delivery of occupational therapy by OTAs who are being supervised by regulated occupational therapists.

Many of the examples provided within the book's content are based on the author's clinical and professional experiences throughout her career, or from information that she learned through presentations and workshops either as a presenter or as a participant. Recognizing that the scenarios do not cover all areas of practice, she nonetheless is optimistic that the processes described will assist readers in applying the material to their individual work situations.

It is the author's intent that the information provided within this book will enable the occupational therapist and OTA optimal collaboration, both to enhance and evolve the profession of occupational therapy and to ensure that clients achieve their best sense of well-being.

References

Canadian Association of Occupational Therapists. (2024). *Competencies for Occupational Therapist Assistants*. Retrieved from: https://caot. ca/document/8146/Competencies%20OTA%20EN%20Feb%208% 202024.pdf

Acknowledgments

I first want to acknowledge Dr. Patricia (Patty) Rigby, an occupational therapist colleague whom I initially met when we both worked in Saskatchewan. Patty was a dear friend and an esteemed colleague, with her research contributing to extensive growth within our occupational therapy profession. After Patty's relocation to work at the University of Toronto, we had the opportunity to reconnect at the 2015 CAOT conference in Winnipeg, Manitoba. I shared my involvement in advocating for increased recognition of OTAs within our profession but was unsure of additional ways to proceed. Patty strongly recommended that I write a book on the OT and OTA collaboration, which was the initial inspiration for this book. Unfortunately, Patty passed away in 2018 resulting in a devastating loss for our profession, and I want to take this opportunity to share how grateful I am for her encouragement to initiate this project.

I am extremely grateful to Sandy Gerber for sharing her expertise in developing effective collaborations through her book *Emotional Magnetism: How to Communicate to Ignite Connection in Your Relationships*. Sandy's description of the four emotional magnets she refers to as Safety, Achievement, Value, and Experience is a productive tool that assists in understanding our decision-making processes and how we interact with others. Sandy's knowledge of communication has been very beneficial to me in growing my personal relationships as well as within my career as an occupational therapist. As is reinforced in my book, building trusting relationships is necessary between occupational therapists and occupational therapist assistants (OTAs) to ensure that effective, safe, and ethical treatments are provided to all clients. Building collaborative relationships in the overall work setting is also necessary to ensure a safe working environment. My experiences over the years working in clinical practice, management, and as an educator for therapist assistants have reinforced that effective communication with clients and families, colleagues, employers, partners such as medical vendors, and students is essential to achieve successful outcomes. After completing Sandy's quiz and learning that my emotional magnet is Safety, I am now more aware of how I approach individuals and groups. Sandy's book has also taught me how to better understand the emotional magnets of others for better connections. Thank-you, Sandy, for this outstanding resource!!

I have been fortunate to collaborate with many OTAs throughout my clinical career, which greatly improved the timely and positive outcomes for clients within our care. I want to acknowledge a specific OTA colleague, Avril McCready-Wirth, who contributed her extensive knowledge and strong skillset in a collaboration to occupational therapy within an acute care hospital setting in Regina, Saskatchewan. The treatments we provided as an occupational therapy team assisted our clients in receiving the treatment they required in an effective, safe, and timely manner within a welcoming environment, and I have included some of these shared experiences within the book. Another recent OTA connection I have developed is with Debra Cooper, an OTA/PTA in Toronto, Ontario. Debra is the Chair of the CAOT OTA/PTA Practice Network and she has made incredible progress in involving OTAs within our profession. She agreed to contribute to Chapter 2, *Developing Trusting Relationships*, from an OTA perspective and I am so appreciative of being able to include her areas of expertise.

I am extremely grateful to my friend Lori Amdam who has shared her healthcare expertise as it pertains to this book and who has been an excellent listener and supporter of this project. My instructor colleagues at Medicine Hat College have provided encouragement and insight throughout this process, and the team at CAOT offered excellent resources and assistance when I needed their guidance.

Last, but definitely not least, is the incredible support I have received from family. My brother Al Gillespie is skilled at writing and has been there when I needed his ideas on topics to include and how they should be presented. My daughters

Jennifer Magotiaux and Tanya Magotiaux, who grew up having to listen to their mom always talking about occupational therapy, provided some excellent thoughts and concepts throughout this process and gave me strong encouragement when I needed it. I am so very grateful for the ongoing support of my husband Jim Morris, who has consistently been there for me since I made the decision to write this book. He gladly offered a second pair of eyes to review my written drafts and make potential alterations from the beginning to the point of completion. Jim's son, Sean Morris, kindly gifted me an author resource, notebook, and pen when I decided to create this book and has continued to regularly check in on my progress. Jim's daughter, Laurie Gardner, consistently provides ongoing support and has been a positive influence throughout this project. I am more than grateful to have such incredible support from my family.

Thank-you to everyone!

Heather Gillespie
Nanaimo, British Columbia, Canada

1

OTA Education, Fieldwork, and Accreditation

Objectives

After completing this chapter, the reader will be able to:

- ♦ Understand the profession of occupational therapy.
- ♦ Recognize the role of occupational therapist assistants (OTAs) in occupational therapy service delivery within rehabilitation.
- ♦ Understand the history of OTA training in Canada.
- ♦ Recognize the foundational knowledge and skills of OTA graduates from an accredited education program.
- ♦ Be aware of culturally safe approaches learned by OTAs during occupational therapy service delivery.
- ♦ Learn of the benefits of intraprofessional education opportunities including fieldwork for both student occupational therapists and OTA students.

Key Terms

- ♦ Occupational therapy
- ♦ Occupational therapist
- ♦ Occupational therapist assistant (OTA)

DOI: 10.4324/9781003498391-1

- ◆ Occupational therapist competencies
- ◆ OTA competencies
- ◆ Cultural safety
- ◆ Accreditation standards
- ◆ OTA knowledge base
- ◆ Clinical practice skills
- ◆ Fieldwork education
- ◆ Role-emerging placements
- ◆ Intraprofessional fieldwork collaboration

Frequently Asked Questions (FAQs) are included at the end of this chapter.

What Is Occupational Therapy?

Occupational therapy is described on the CAOT website as "a type of health care that helps to solve the problems that interfere with a person's ability to do the things that are important to them" (CAOT, 2024a). It promotes health, well-being, and quality of life by supporting access to, initiation of, and sustained participation in the things that clients want and need to do in their daily life, with the people and in the places that they want to participate in these occupations (Egan and Restall, 2022). Those working within the diverse occupational therapy profession assist clients of all ages and health status, who are experiencing or are possibly at risk of experiencing difficulties participating in their daily activities. A master's degree in occupational therapy is the minimal educational requirement for entry-level education in Canada for occupational therapists.

Occupational therapy is a healthcare profession that is not clearly understood by the general public or by many other healthcare disciplines, managers, and employers within Canada. The author's extensive clinical experience and numerous communications with colleagues over the years has indicated that the term "occupational therapy" is often met with confusion, along with the question "What does that mean?" Clients have expressed concern about what their occupational therapy treatment will be, many believing it has to do with jobs within the context of the word "occupation." This may also result in a panic reaction by older adults who frequently respond by saying "I don't want to find a job – I have worked all of my life and now I am retired." This can result in some clients declining occupational therapy treatment based on their interpretation of the meaning of "occupation." Although initial occupational therapy was associated with work, the profession has diversified into several different practice areas. A clear explanation by the occupational therapist of the current significance and meaning of the term "occupation" as it relates to the therapy will provide clarity for the client and caregivers in increasing their understanding and how it will potentially assist them in meeting their needs. This transparency will also assist the client or substitute decision-maker to feel comfortable providing informed consent that is required to proceed with assessment and treatment planning.

It is also important to explain the occupational therapist's role to the clients, including regulation if they reside in a Canadian province, and to discuss their collaboration with occupational therapist assistants within their work environment.

Occupational Therapist Assistants (OTAs) – Who Are They?

Literature reviews over the past 20 years indicate that the role of occupational therapist assistants (OTAs), or support personnel, continues to be an important component in clients' ability to access occupational therapy, as well as to ensure cost-effectiveness.

- ◆ Occupational therapists must use innovative strategies, including developing partnerships with support personnel, to promote occupational therapy service delivery through improving accessibility and cost-effectiveness (von Zweck & Gillespie, 1998, p. 60).
- ◆ OTAs and occupational therapists working together can provide safe and quality care in economically uncertain healthcare environments (Blake, Park, & Brice-Leddy, 2015, p. 14).

◆ "With heavy workloads and an ongoing need for quick patient discharges from hospital, occupational therapists benefit from working with occupational therapist assistants (OTAs) to allow them more time for assessments and discharge planning" (Vo & Feenstra, 2015, p. 23).

◆ Early supportive discharge for complex neurology rehab patients through "collaboration with home care teams, and in particular the delegation of rehabilitation tasks to rehabilitation assistants, is elegantly simple but hugely effective" (Blandford, 2018, p. 29).

However, there needs to be an increased understanding by occupational therapists, practice leaders, and therapy managers of the skills and knowledge that OTAs bring to clinical practice. Occupational therapists need to feel confident in involving OTAs appropriately in client intervention programs. OTAs also need to understand their role and that they are accountable to the supervising occupational therapist when delivering client interventions.

The changes within our economic and political environments which are resulting in noticeable differences to the provision of Canadian healthcare, including rehabilitation, are forcing our profession to be open to alternative ways of delivering occupational therapy more cost-effectively, while ensuring that our clients receive efficient and ethical care. One approach to achieving this is through consistently involving OTAs in service delivery to enhance clients' engagement in occupations.

The World Federation of Occupational Therapists (WFOT) 2019 Position Statement, *Occupational Therapy and Rehabilitation*, states that:

Occupational therapy has a substantial role in rehabilitation due to its:

◆ Appreciation of rehabilitation as a human right
◆ Person centred approach
◆ Expertise in understanding the complex interactions between the person/family/community, the environment and occupations

- ◆ Main goal being occupational engagement and full participation; and,
- ◆ Cost effectiveness for society.

(WFOT, 2019, p. 1)

This role can be augmented through building an effective occupational therapist and OTA collaboration in more work settings throughout the country.

Who are occupational therapist assistants or OTAs? On their website the Canadian Occupational Therapist Assistant and Physical Therapist Assistant Educators Council (or COPEC) states, "Occupational therapist assistants, or OTAs, work under the direction and supervision of occupational therapists to deliver assigned occupational therapy services. They work with clients on a one-to-one basis or in groups, to engage these individuals in meaningful activities, focusing on compensatory or remedial treatment interventions to either learn or re-learn how to achieve optimal independence and reducing barriers to function" (Canadian Occupational Therapist Assistant and Physical Therapist Assistant Educators Council, 2023).

However, as there is no regulation for OTAs in Canada and therefore no protection of title, it can be challenging to understand an OTA's role in some environments. They can be identified in various ways such as support personnel, rehabilitation assistants, rehabilitation aides, occupational therapy assistants, OTA/PTAs – and the list goes on. The lack of protected title increases the confusion concerning an individual's skills and knowledge. These can vary from someone who was trained "on-the-job" many years ago, to an internationally educated occupational therapist awaiting substantial equivalency to practice in Canada, to a graduate of a previous OTA/PTA certificate education program, to a graduate of a current accredited therapist assistant diploma education program. The role of an OTA can also be taken on by kinesiologists in private clinics, education assistants in the school system, or driver instructors in Driver Rehab programs on the condition that the therapy treatments they are providing have been assigned by a supervising occupational therapist who is accountable for the treatment being provided.

Although there is no regulatory protection of title, it is encouraged through the Canadian Association of Occupational Therapists (CAOT) that the designation "occupational therapist assistant or OTA" be used more consistently because this identification reinforces their main role which is to assist the supervising occupational therapist in the delivery of occupational therapy treatments. CAOT includes this title within their website (CAOT, 2024a) and it is used in the updated CAOT competency document: *Competencies for Occupational Therapist Assistants* (CAOT, 2024b). A similar title is referenced within the Canadian Physiotherapy Association (CPA), with the designation "physiotherapist assistant or PTA" being included on their website (CPA, 2024). Other titles such as rehabilitation assistants, rehab aides, or support personnel can be confusing within certain environments because it may be unclear which healthcare professional has assigned specific client treatments and therefore who is responsible for the required supervision.

The variability in OTA-related education and training leads to discrepancies and confusion in occupational therapists' understanding of their abilities and knowledge as the therapists often do not know "what they're getting" when a new OTA is hired. This results in a lack of confidence among many occupational therapists in involving OTAs in client care, which in turn can create a strain on their working relationships within the profession.

Employers, managers, and practice leaders within healthcare settings also demonstrate misunderstandings of the OTA roles due to the variety of educational experiences, skills, and career backgrounds with which OTAs enter their work environments. This can often result in further challenges when involving OTAs in occupational therapy service delivery.

Evolution of OTA Education

Occupational therapist assistants have been involved in occupational therapy service delivery since 1953 when an education program was initiated at the Kingston Psychiatric Hospital in Ontario to train assistants to work in psychiatric hospitals in Ontario. This program existed until 1971 (Salvatori, 2001).

During the 1960s, an on-the-job training model was emerging in several rehabilitation settings in Canada (Salvatori, 2001). On-the-job training refers to a hands-on method of teaching skills needed to perform a specific job. An occupational therapist with access to an OTA (or support personnel as they were referred to at that time) would be responsible for teaching support personnel certain skills related to the occupational therapy treatment they would be assigned for a specific client. Each occupational therapist may have had a unique approach to that treatment, requiring the support personnel to learn and regularly adapt to each occupational therapist's individual method and approach. Many occupational therapists agreed with this style of support personnel learning as they had control of what skills were taught and the specific knowledge the support personnel were given. The negative outcome was the lack of uniformity in training within practice settings and across the country.

CAOT did recognize an aide and an assistant as two levels of support personnel in the late 1970s. The aides would be on-the-job trained and a 12-month training program was recommended for assistants (Salvatori, 2001, p. 221). The Discussion Paper on the Role and use of Support Personnel in the Rehabilitation Disciplines (1989) was generated by CAOT along with the Canadian Physiotherapy Association and the Canadian Association of Speech Language Pathology and Audiology (1989). The recommendations within this discussion paper included:

- ◆ Maximal use of support personnel
- ◆ Therapists must supervise the support personnel
- ◆ The type and amount of supervision is determined by the supervisor
- ◆ Support personnel could not interpret referrals, provide initial assessments, interpret findings, plan or modify treatments, chart, discuss confidential information with client or family or plan discharge
- ◆ On-the-job training following basic skill acquisition
- ◆ Differing scope of practice from existing disciplines
- ◆ Service delivery and training model evaluations

(Salvatori, 2001, p. 221)

The inclusion of support personnel in rehabilitation care delivery was considered to result in expanded services and decreased healthcare costs but concerns were expressed that there would be increased risk of harm to clients, conflict in roles, ethical and legal implications, availability of therapists to supervise, and limited employment opportunities for the support personnel (Salvatori, 2020, p. 221).

These discussions initiated further conversations related to formal education programs, resulting in the first rehabilitation assistants graduating in Kelowna, British Columbia, in 1991 with a certificate qualification (Salvatori, 2001, p. 222). In 1992, Humber College in Toronto, Ontario, initiated a part-time program for OTAs currently working in the field and followed up with implementing a full-time program the following year (Salvatori, 2001, p. 222).

The report on the Role and Use of Support Personnel in the Rehabilitation Disciplines by Hagler and colleagues from the University of Alberta was released in 1993, and the responses from those interviewed indicated that support personnel need to be supervised by therapists and that "they preferred a training model that combined practical experiences with academic instruction" (Salvatori, 2001, p. 222). CAOT responded to the Hagler report listing some concerns including the methodology used in the study, and said that they could support a "formal training program for assistants if it was generic in nature, no longer than one year in duration, and did not require a fieldwork component" (Salvatori, 2001, p. 222). CAOT did agree with the report's stating that support personnel needed to be supervised by an occupational therapist. Hagler, Madill, and Kennedy (1994) responded to CAOT with clarifications surrounding the methodology used within the study, and agreed that it is not only the occupational therapist's responsibility to supervise the support personnel but it is "incumbent upon the employers, clinical administrators, programme supervisors, clinical professionals, and support workers themselves to ensure that support workers do not provide occupational therapy services without supervision by an occupational therapist" (Hagler, Madill, & Kennedy, 1994, p. 216). In response to CAOT's reference to the formal education programs, it was stated that interviews during the Hagler study indicated that "1) more training was considered desirable, 2) certain knowledge and skill areas specific to occupational therapy were considered important, and 3) if future support workers were trained in this way, they could provide more assistance to occupational therapists" (Hagler, Madill, & Kennedy, 1994, p. 217). They also argued that fieldwork is necessary within the education programs to improve service delivery, stating that "a classroom educated and clinic-trained occupational therapy support worker would hit the ground running" (Hagler, Madill, & Kennedy, 1994, p. 218).

The next step taken by CAOT was forming a task force in 1995 to review the relationship of occupational therapy support personnel to CAOT (von Zweck & Gillespie, 1998). It was recognized that there was a need to effectively define support personnel roles and be involved in planning and developing their education programs which would assist in improving occupational therapy services across the country (von Zweck & Gillespie, 1998). A revised position statement on Support Personnel in Occupational Therapy Services (CAOT, 1988) was one of the outcomes from the Task Force recommendations and provided new directions for CAOT related to support personnel in Canada. Occupational therapy support personnel were defined within the position statement as "any workers who are not qualified occupational therapists but are knowledgeable in the field of occupational therapy through education and training and are directly involved in the provision of occupational therapy services under the supervision of an occupational therapist" (CAOT, 1998, p. 112). Additionally, it stated that the support personnels' skills and knowledge "may be obtained through a formalized training program which is based on a validated competency profile for occupational therapy support personnel" (CAOT, 1998, p.111). Recommendations for the requirements to be included in these education programs were described in the position statement, including "preparing the students for entry level practice as a support worker in occupational therapy through academic and fieldwork education" (CAOT, 1998, p. 111) and that, as regards fieldwork experiences, if "supervised by qualified occupational therapists or at the discretion of the supervising occupational therapist and educational facility faculty, these duties may be shared with appropriately trained and competent support personnel" (CAOT, 1998, p. 111). It is also interesting to note that the position statement recommends that "distance education methods be available where possible to access the curriculum" (CAOT, 1998, p. 111), with distance education being defined as "the use of alternate teaching methods which allow the learner to participate at locations or at times which are convenient to them through correspondence programs, computer on-line courses, teleconferencing, video conferencing and block scheduling of practical sessions" (CAOT, 1998, p. 112). Distance education or distributed learning therapist assistant programs are currently available in certain education colleges within Canada.

Coinciding with CAOT's development of resources and tools relating to support personnel based on the Task Force recommendations, there were more certificate programs initiated at educational institutions across the country – some were discipline-specific OTA or PTA, and others were combined OTA and PTA programs. The content of the programs included both theoretical and practical knowledge, as well as fieldwork placements. The number of fieldwork hours required by each program varied across the country.

In the mid 1990s–2000, many education programs advanced from a certificate program to a two-year diploma program, and this continues to be the current recommended length for therapist assistant education programs in Canada.

The Canadian Occupational Therapist Assistant and Physiotherapist Education Council (COPEC) was formed due to the growing number of publicly funded college education programs in Canada in the mid- to late 1990s. The main goals of COPEC are that members share best practices and resources, and liaise with provincial organizations on matters relating to therapist assistants. The COPEC website http://copec.ca/ contains information on the group's history, resources for educators as well as for OTA/PTAs in Canada, useful contacts, and news and events.

OTA/PTA Education Accreditation

As a result of the diversity of the therapist assistant education programs causing confusion as to the knowledge and skills of graduating OTAs and PTAs, the Occupational Therapist Assistant and Physiotherapist Assistant Education Accreditation Program, or OTA & PTA EAP, was initiated in 2009 with two pilot accreditation reviews occurring in early 2012 (Davidson, 2015, p. 11). The accreditation process includes submission of a Self Study Report by the education program with an off-site review of the report by the Peer Review Team and an on-site review of the education program (Davidson, 2015, p. 11).

The Occupational Therapist Assistant & Physiotherapist Assistant Education Accreditation Program (or OTA & PTA EAP) is governed by both Physiotherapy Education Accreditation Canada (PEAC) and the Canadian Association of Occupational Therapists (CAOT), (OTA & PTA EAP, 2013). The accreditation process is currently voluntary and is open to publicly and privately funded programs. Although most of the accredited programs are combined OTA and PTA, there is an option for single discipline programs to be accredited. Of note, Quebec is not included in the EAP as their educational system is different from the other programs in Canada.

Occupational therapists working within regulated provinces are legally liable for the therapy services provided by OTAs, and therefore need the assistants to be "capable and safe in the delivery of care, and assistants need clear communication during the assignment of tasks, which should be appropriate to their skills" (Douglas, 2018, p. 6). Accreditation of the education programs from which OTAs graduate plays a key role in "promoting effective work among occupational therapists and OTAs and will benefit the clients we serve" (Douglas, 2018, p. 6). The accreditation process explores the components of an education program including the curriculum, appropriate resources including learning materials and equipment within practical lab spaces, and OTA fieldwork placement requirements. The OTA components of an accredited education program must be instructed by an occupational therapist and the PTA components must be taught by a physiotherapist (Douglas, 2018, p. 6).

Although accreditation of formal education programs is currently voluntary, many healthcare organizations are now including graduation from an accredited OTA and PTA education program as a requirement for employment. This provides occupational therapists and employers, managers, and leaders, in all work settings, with a stronger and consistent understanding of the basic knowledge and skills learned by an OTA during their education.

The OTA & PTA EAP website www.otapta.ca provides the current accreditation status of specific programs opting for accreditation, (OTA & PTA EAP, 2013).

The four main functions of accreditation as described in the 2018 Accreditation Standards document are to:

1. Establish standards, criteria, policies and procedures for the evaluation of occupational therapist assistant and physiotherapist assistant education programs.
2. Conduct assessments that encourage institutions to maintain and improve their programs.
3. Determine compliance with established criteria for accreditation.
4. Provide ongoing consultation to occupational therapist assistant and physiotherapist assistant education programs.

(OTA & PTA EAP, 2018, p. 6)

The OTA & PTA EAP Peer Review Team (PRT) consists of the following members:

- ◆ An occupational therapist representing CAOT
- ◆ An occupational therapist who is an OTA educator
- ◆ A physiotherapist representing PEAC
- ◆ A physiotherapist who is a PTA educator

As of 2019, the decision was made that if two OTA/PTA educators cannot be recruited for the PRT, "one of the two educators will be replaced with a team member with relevant OTA/PTA practice or education experience" (retrieved from: https://otapta.ca/english/get-involved/become-a-peer-review-team-member.php).

The responsibilities of the members of the PRT are to:

◆ Complete a preliminary and site review of an OTA & PTA education program.
◆ Verify and supplement evidence provided by the education program in the Self Study Report.
◆ Assess the program within the context of its environment.
◆ Prepare and submit a report about the program's compliance with the OTA & PTA EAP accreditation standards (OTA & PTA EAP, 2020, p. 51).

The accreditation standards document includes five standards common to both OTA and PTA:

◆ Standard 1: The Educational Program and Its Environment
◆ Standard 2: Faculty
◆ Standard 3: Students
◆ Standard 4: Program Evaluation
◆ Standard 5: Accountability

Standard 6 is divided into Standard 6 OTA and Standard 6 PTA and the standards are adapted from the competency profiles of each profession which includes the CAOT *Practice Profile for Support Personnel in Occupational Therapy 2009* and the NPAG *Essential Competency Profile for Physiotherapist Assistants in Canada 2012* (OTA & PTA EAP, 2018, pp. 8–9).

It is necessary to note here that the CAOT *Practice Profile* has recently been updated to the *Competencies for Occupational Therapist Assistants 2024*. The decision to proceed with this document revision was based on the new *Competencies for Occupational Therapists in Canada* (*COTC*) document that was published in November 2021. The updated 2024 competencies will be referred to throughout the remainder of this book, but as they have only recently been published, they have not yet been incorporated into the OTA & PTA education accreditation standards. Therefore, the 2009 *Practice Profile* for OTAs will be referenced in this section.

It is essential for occupational therapists who are involving OTAs within their clinical practice to understand the learning they have achieved during their OTA education programs. Due to the accreditation process being voluntary, the therapist needs to confirm with each OTA whether they graduated from an accredited or non-accredited education program (this will be discussed further in Chapter 2). If the OTA did graduate from an accredited education program, the entry-level competencies within Standard 6 *Occupational Therapist Assistant Competencies* are described here to provide further evidence to occupational therapists as to the OTAs' knowledge.

Role OTA 6.1 Communicator

The program prepares students to use effective communication to develop and maintain appropriate and respectful relationships with clients, families, care providers, and other stakeholders.

Criterion

♦ **OTA 6.1.1**: Engages in and facilitates effective verbal and nonverbal communication with the client, supervising occupational therapist and interprofessional team members.

♦ **OTA 6.1.2**: Utilizes objective and effective written communication skills with the client, supervising occupational therapist and interprofessional team members.

♦ **OTA 6.1.3**: Supports diversity in communication by using strategies to reduce communication barriers with different populations in different practice contexts and incorporates sensitive practice.

Role OTA 6.2 Collaborator

The program prepares students to work collaboratively and effectively within an interprofessional team and with others to achieve optimal client care.

Criterion

- ◆ **OTA 6.2.1**: Supports collaboration with the client, supervising occupational therapist and interprofessional team members.
- ◆ **OTA 6.2.2**: Participates actively as an interprofessional team member.
- ◆ **OTA 6.2.3**: Anticipates, identifies, prevents and resolves conflict.

Role OTA 6.3 Effective Practitioner

The program prepares students to manage time, prioritize competing priorities in collaboration with occupational therapists and support the delivery of effective and efficient practice.

Criterion

- ◆ **OTA 6.3.1**: Manages activities that support effective service delivery and integrated client care.
- ◆ **OTA 6.3.2**: Uses human, financial, and physical resources effectively.
- ◆ **OTA 6.3.3**: Recognizes, respects, and participates in established organizational quality improvement activities.

Role OTA 6.4 Change Agent/Advocate

The program prepares students to understand how to responsibly use knowledge and influence within their role to promote the health and well-being of individual clients, communities and populations.

Criterion

- ◆ **OTA 6.4.1**: Promotes the benefits and value of their professional group.
- ◆ **OTA 6.4.2**: Assists clients in making life changes in support of their health goals as determined by the supervising occupational therapist.
- ◆ **OTA 6.4.3**: Considers the impact of the determinants of health on the well-being of clients served.

Role OTA 6.5 Reflective Practitioner

The program prepares students to incorporate critique, reflection, and quality improvement in their everyday practice and through lifelong learning.

Criterion

- ◆ **OTA 6.5.1**: Recognizes the need for professional development through reflective practices and self-directed lifelong learning.
- ◆ **OTA 6.5.2**: Modifies service delivery based on personal reflection and external feedback under the supervision of the occupational therapist.
- ◆ **OTA 6.5.3**: Supports the supervising occupational therapist in applying an evidenceinformed approach in their services.

Role OTA 6.6 Professional Practitioner

The program prepares students to commit to the best interests of clients and society through ethical and legal practice and high personal standards of behavior.

Criterion

- ◆ **OTA 6.6.1**: Demonstrates ethical behavior with clients and team members in a variety of situations.
- ◆ **OTA 6.6.2**: Respects diversity and demonstrates sensitive practice.
- ◆ **OTA 6.6.3**: Maintains personal and professional boundaries.
- ◆ **OTA 6.6.4**: Performs within the limits of personal competence within their own professional scope.

Role OTA 6.7 Educated Practitioner in Enabling Occupation

The program prepares students to be skilled practitioners in enabling occupation using evidence-based processes that focus on a client's occupations – including self-care, productive pursuits, and leisure – as a medium for action and outcome during performance of assigned tasks and within established guidelines and limits.

Criterion

- ◆ **OTA 6.7.1**: Safely and efficiently supports the occupational therapist who is the expert in enabling occupation.
- ◆ **OTA 6.7.2**: Works to enable occupation with specific populations and occupational performance issues in a range of practice contexts.
- ◆ **OTA 6.7.3**: Gathers information and data related to the client's status as assigned by the occupational therapist.
- ◆ **OTA 6.7.4**: Implements the interventions assigned by the occupational therapist.
- ◆ **OTA 6.7.5**: Demonstrates effective problem solving and judgment related to assigned service components.
- ◆ **OTA 6.7.6**: Participates in the learning process for clients, team members, peers, students and any other learners within their service.

(OTA & PTA EAP, 2018, pp. 44–58)

Updated Occupational Therapy Competencies

As mentioned earlier in this chapter, a new document on *Competencies for Occupational Therapists in Canada (COTC)* was published in November 2021. These are included within the provincial regulation requirements for occupational therapists and are being incorporated into their education programs.

Within this new document, the following competencies were created within Domain A (*Occupational Therapy Expertise*) and Domain F (*Engagement with the Profession*):

The competent occupational therapist is expected to:

- ◆ **A7 Manage the assignment of services to assistants and others**
  - • **A7.1** Identify practice situations where clients may benefit from services assigned to assistants or others.

- **A7.2** Assign services only to assistants and others who are competent to deliver the services.
- **A7.3** Monitor the safety and effectiveness of assignments through supervision, mentoring, teaching, and coaching.
- **A7.4** Follow the regulatory guidance for assigning and supervising services.

(ACOTRO, ACOTUP, CAOT, 2021, p. 11)

◆ **F2 Show leadership in the workplace**
F2.1 Support assistants, students, support staff, volunteers, and other team members.

(ACOTRO, ACOTUP, CAOT, 2021, p. 17)

Based on these new occupational therapist competencies, an increased understanding of collaborating with OTAs needs to be a component of each therapist's role in clinical practice or within their responsibilities as a leader, manager, or employer of occupational therapists and OTAs. It will also be essential that student occupational therapists learn about the therapist and OTA relationship within their master's education programs.

As noted earlier, the Practice Profile has now been replaced with the *Competencies for Occupational Therapist Assistants 2024*. This document aligns with the occupational therapist competencies within the COTC, providing a needed consistency within the occupational therapy profession (CAOT, 2024b). The meaning of the term *competency* in occupational therapy as described by WFOT includes "an integration of individual behaviours that are measurable and are critical to the practice of occupational therapy; knowledge regarding occupational therapy concepts, theories, and processes; and personal values and attitudes that enable effective occupational therapy work performance. Competencies focus on what can be learned, demonstrated, and measured in order to have capacity for safe and effective occupational therapy practice" (WFOT, 2022, p.1). The competencies described in the new document reflect a broad range of OTA skills and abilities. These skills and abilities are to be required and interpreted as to the supervising occupational therapist's assignments to the

OTAs. All of these competencies will not necessarily be included in everyday practice (CAOT, 2024b).

Education Trends

Education trends in current OTA/PTA diploma education programs provide a greater depth of curriculum content compared to the initial certificate programs and they continue to emphasize the integration of theoretical and hands-on or practical training. Realistic scenarios are provided to the students and certain education programs have hired standardized participants to role-play clients with specific conditions. The students can then practice clinical skills they have learned by providing treatment to these "clients" using appropriate equipment and assistive devices.

Examples of some of these clinical skills are:

1. Students can incorporate their knowledge about the multiple wheelchair options currently available in the medical equipment market and complete hands-on adjustments required in order to ensure appropriate fit of a wheelchair for a particular "client". This practice assists in building their competence in using various tools for making required adjustments and adding appropriate adaptations or pieces of equipment to the wheelchairs. This also provides the opportunity for students to see both manual and power-operated wheelchairs of various sizes, in addition to the extensive variety of cushions and back supports that are available.
2. They can also practice teaching exercises or activities to the "clients" using principles they have learned within their courses. One example is the "tell me, show me, watch me do it" principle. They begin this process with telling the "client" how to do the task, as well as explaining why they will be doing it. The OTA will also reinforce what not to do, particularly if it is a safety concern. The next step is that the OTA student will demonstrate how to do the task and, again, reinforcing the safest way to

proceed. The final part of this teaching process is watching the "client" perform the task. OTAs are encouraged to observe and resist helping out if the "client" is missing a step, as this will enable decision-making and problem-solving resulting in more effective learning.

The inclusion of real-life case scenarios within the OTA education programs contributes to the students' learning about critical thinking, a component of clinical reasoning. They must incorporate problem-solving processes within these case studies to provide the best and safest treatments to the "clients" that will assist in meeting their goals. This process being included within their education increases their confidence and provides experiences that they can incorporate as needed when treating actual clients within their fieldwork placements and as they begin their careers.

It is also important to inform the OTA students that there may be certain situations while treating clients in which they may feel uncomfortable or unsafe, and it is important to be as prepared as possible in these circumstances. These instances could include:

1. The OTA has been asked to assist a male client who recently experienced quadriplegia following a motor vehicle accident to learn self-care skills including dressing himself. The client and the OTA are both aged in their early twenties. In this situation, the OTA and/or the client may be uncomfortable with the client needing to be unclothed to proceed with this treatment. If aware of this possibility ahead of time, the OTA can assure the client that they are aware this may be an uncomfortable situation, but the outcome will be an increase in his self-care independence.

2. The OTA has been asked to assist a client with relearning cooking tasks within a mental health setting. The client was admitted to the facility due to substance abuse and has improved to a level that discharge home is being planned. The client enjoys baking and the OTA decides to have the client make a cake following a simple recipe. The client initially keeps to the directions, but then forgets

to add a necessary ingredient. The OTA cues the client about the missing ingredient, but the client disagrees, stating that they have added the ingredient, and starts to become angry. In preparation for this incident possibly occurring, the OTA needs to know how to deescalate the situation and also to ensure that any sharp utensils, including knives, are not closely accessible to the client. During the treatment it would also be beneficial to have near by a colleague who can assist as needed.

These are only a couple of examples of uncomfortable and/or unsafe situations that may occur during client treatments, and OTA students need to be aware of them and provide options for planning ahead as much as possible.

An additional education trend is a commitment to fostering interprofessional and intraprofessional collaboration within the curriculum. The need for incorporating intraprofessional student learning was stated by Salvatori: "Shared learning experiences for both professional entry-level and assistant level students would facilitate the development of collaborative relationships prior to entering practice" (Salvatori, 2001, p. 226). This was reinforced by Jung and colleagues: "There is clearly a need not only to define roles and responsibilities of those involved in providing occupational therapy services but also to educate students at the professional and assistant level for future collaborative practice" (Jung, Salvatori, & Martin, 2008, p. 42). Fieldwork placements are an integral component in all programs to provide experience with these collaborations, and although there are no requirements as to specific settings or forms of collaboration that a therapist assistant student needs to complete within fieldwork placements, the education programs attempt to provide each student with experience in as varied clinical settings as is possible.

There are increasing numbers of OTA/PTA education programs being established within Canada, although we are unable to know the specific statistics. This is due to accreditation of OTA/PTA education programs currently being a voluntary option and there is also no database of all therapist assistant education programs being offered in the country.

Cultural Safety

A further revision to education content is based on recent updates related to the work of the Truth and Reconciliation Commission including the effects of colonization. This has led to an increased understanding of the atrocities that took place in residential schools in addition to an improved acknowledgment of inequities and diversity occurring within our society. This has resulted in the subject of cultural sensitivity awareness while working with Indigenous populations and other cultures being better incorporated into healthcare education curricula. Cultural safety is needed within healthcare and is based on respectful engagement that addresses power imbalances, often resulting from racism and discrimination. Culturally safe environments result in people from all cultures feeling protected when receiving healthcare services.

Learning about cultural safety is imperative within healthcare education programs. This includes understanding cultural humility, which is a self-reflection of one's biases and systemic beliefs. Once there is increased personal awareness of these issues, learning about more effective approaches while working with clients from all cultures, including Indigenous Peoples, will result in improved therapeutic relationships and more effective outcomes for those needing occupational therapy and other healthcare services (Government of Canada, 2016).

As defined in the 2024 *Competencies for Occupational Therapist Assistants*, the term "culturally 'safer' is a refinement to the concept of cultural safety. Competent OTAs do everything they can to provide culturally safe care, but they remain aware they are in a position of power in relation to clients. They are mindful that many marginalized people – Indigenous people for example – have a history of serious mistreatment in healthcare settings. These clients may never feel fully safe. OTAs allow those who receive the service to determine what they consider to be safe. They support them in drawing strength from their identity, culture, and community. Because cultural safety is unlikely to be fully achievable, we work toward it" (CAOT, 2024b, pp. 13–14).

As previously stated, the Competencies for OTAs are based on the *Competencies for Occupational Therapists in Canada* or COTC (ACOTRO, ACOTUP, CAOT, 2021). The COTC "acknowledged the presence and impact of systemic racism in Canada which has great meaning for the role that the competencies have in shifting the practice of occupational therapy" (CAOT, 2024b, p. 3).

OTA Competencies and indicators within Domain C, *Culture, Equity, and Justice*, state the following:

The competent OTA is expected to:

◆ **C1 Promote equity in practice**
  - **C1.1** Identify the ongoing effects of colonization and settlement on occupational opportunities and services for Indigenous Peoples.
  - **C1.2** Analyze the effects of systemic and historical factors on people, groups, and their *occupational possibilities*.
  - **C1.3** Challenge biases and social structures that privilege or marginalize people and communities.
  - **C1.4** Respond to the social, structural, political, and ecological determinants of health, wellbeing, and occupational opportunities.
  - **C1.5** Work to reduce the effects of the unequal distribution of power and resources on the delivery of occupational therapy services.
  - **C1.6** Support the factors that promote health, wellbeing and occupations.
◆ **C2 Promote anti-oppressive behaviour and culturally safer, inclusive relationships**
  - **C2.1** Contribute to a practice environment that is culturally safer, anti-racist, anti-ableist, and inclusive.
  - **C2.2** Practise self-awareness to minimize personal bias and inequitable behaviour based on *social position and power*.
  - **C2.3** Demonstrate respect and *humility* when engaging with clients and integrate their

understanding of health, wellbeing, healing, and occupation into the service plan.

- **C2.4** Seek out resources to help develop culturally safer and inclusive approaches.
- **C2.5** Collaborate with local partners, such as interpreters and leaders.

◆ **C3 Contribute to equitable access to** occupational participation **and occupational therapy**

- **C3.1** Raise clients' awareness of the role of and the right to occupation.
- **C3.2** Facilitate clients' participation in occupations supporting health and wellbeing.
- **C3.3** Assist with access to support networks and resources.
- **C3.4** Navigate systemic barriers to support clients and self.
- **C3.5** Engage in critical dialogue with other interested parties on social injustices and inequitable opportunities for occupations.
- **C3.6** Advocate for environments and policies that support sustainable occupational participation.
- **C3.7** Raise awareness of limitations and bias in data, information, and systems.

(CAOT, 2024b, p. 9)

These competencies will guide the knowledge and skills that OTA students will learn related to culture, equity, and justice within their education programs. One of the first topics to discuss is cultural humility by asking students to reflect on who they are, their cultural perspectives, and their possible biases. This will initiate the process of increasing their understanding of their own feelings and appreciation that all clients, as human beings, need to be treated the same.

A general clinical practice approach that OTA students can learn about is how to initiate communication with clients and/or family members with whom they will be working. They can open the conversation by introducing themselves to the client and/or family members and explain their role as an OTA and the treatment(s) they plan to provide with the client's or family member's consent. This introduction would also include the name of the supervising occupational therapist who had assigned the treatment to the OTA.

An additional question that can be asked by the OTA is one recently shared with the author by an occupational therapist colleague who stated that they ask their clients this question when developing their therapeutic relationship:

"Is there something about your culture that could affect your healing that I should know about?"

This type of question demonstrates "cultural safety's broad perspective on 'culture' which is inclusive of socially constructed categories, including ethnicity, gender, ability and socioeconomic status" (Gerlach, 2012, p. 154). It reveals to the client that the OTA recognizes and respects the client's rights related to their cultural safety (Gerlach, 2012, p. 152).

The *Joint Position Statement – Toward Equity and Justice: Enacting an Intersectional Approach to Social Accountability in Occupational Therapy* was recently developed by three Canadian occupational therapy associations: the Canadian Association of Occupational Therapists, the Association of Canadian Occupational Therapy Regulatory Organizations, and the Association of Canadian Occupational Therapy University Programs (CAOT, ACOTRO, ACOTUP, 2024). Those that work in healthcare, including occupational therapists and OTAs, have experienced harm and racism during clinical practice, and this also applies to people who are receiving occupational therapy services (CAOT, ACOTRO, ACOTUP, 2024). OTAs have also reported situations where they have experienced marginalization and estrangement in their workplaces (Penner, Snively, Packham, Henderson, Principi, & Malstrom, 2020). The joint position statement document "justifies and supports actions in occupational therapy to decentre whiteness, address health inequities, and promote occupational participation" and the document asks "occupational therapists, occupational therapist assistants, student occupational therapists, and student occupational therapist assistants to envision an occupational therapy profession that is rooted in social justice, centres equity, and commits to socially accountable principles, processes, and practices" (CAOT, ACOTRO, ACOTUP, 2024, p. 3). Social accountability requires that people who have been historically excluded from discussions and decision making must now be invited to participate in discussions, and that transparency and access to information is available to inform individual, group, and community participation. This is in partnership with those responsible for change being accountable for decisions made, which will likely result in more successful outcomes (CAOT, ACOTRO, ACOTUP, 2024).

The joint position statement document provides guiding recommendations to initiate these changes, and a few of these recommendations include:

◆ Occupational therapist assistants and occupational therapist assistant students, in collaboration with occupational therapists:

- Become familiar with and identify examples of social accountability, intersectionality, oppressions, white supremacy, microaggressions, implicit bias, privilege, cultural humility, culturally safer relationships, and trauma-informed care.
  (CAOT, ACOTRO, ACOTUP, 2024, p. 9)

This recommendation needs to be incorporated within the OTA curriculum to increase this understanding prior to initiating fieldwork placements if possible. This knowledge can then be applied to the clients they will be working with during placements and will better prepare them for initiating their career as an OTA.

- Support co-creation with clients, service users, families, and others within intervention sessions and support equity and social accountability initiatives in the workplace.
  (CAOT, ACOTRO, ACOTUP, 2024, p. 9)

This recommendation should be incorporated into OTA fieldwork placements to increase students' awareness and understanding of supporting clients that they can then apply to their work settings following graduation.

◆ Education:

- Create accessible occupational therapy programs with varied delivery options to meet diverse access needs (e.g. part-time, online, and weekend programs, virtual and in-person fieldwork placements) that can be delivered with and in underserved communities.
  (CAOT, ACOTRO, ACOTUP, 2024, p. 11)

This recommendation applies to both occupational therapist and occupational therapist assistant education programs. There are currently OTA education programs that are delivered online and can be completed on a part-time basis, but this type of accessibility does need to increase across the country and particularly to enable those in remote communities to access this education without needing to relocate.

- Provide relationship-building resources so that all occupational therapy students can engage in fieldwork in settings with current or historical experiences of oppression within the context of developing ethical and reconciliatory long-term community-university (*college*) partnerships.
  (CAOT, ACOTRO, ACOTUP, 2024, p. 12)

This recommendation would apply to fieldwork experiences for both student occupational therapists and OTA students, and potentially within role-emerging placements and/or collaborative intraprofessional fieldwork experiences (discussed in more detail later in this chapter).

OTA Curriculum and Fieldwork

Foundational Knowledge within the OTA Curriculum

Within the diploma level programs, foundational knowledge courses prepare students for profession specific learning. These are samples of courses that are required, although it is important to note that courses will vary within different programs:

- ◆ Anatomy
- ◆ Physiology
- ◆ Psychology
- ◆ Diseases and conditions
- ◆ Health care and rehabilitation
- ◆ OTA and PTA general roles and responsibilities
- ◆ Safe body mechanics
- ◆ Interpersonal communication skills
- ◆ Health care terminology
- ◆ Ethics and professionalism
- ◆ Cultural safety

Core Occupational Therapy Knowledge

General occupational therapy information that OTA students learn in a diploma education program includes but is not limited to:

- ◆ Current occupational therapy theories and ethics
- ◆ Role of the occupational therapist as an OTA supervisor
- ◆ Communication skills with clients and with supervising occupational therapists
- ◆ Therapeutic treatments
- ◆ Intervention principles
- ◆ Critical thinking
- ◆ Activity analysis
- ◆ Grading and adapting theories and processes
- ◆ Principles of teaching
- ◆ Mental health concepts
- ◆ Clinical documentation
- ◆ Occupational participation

- Clinical groups across the lifespan
- Culture, equity, and justice

Clinical Practice Skills

The knowledge and skills that that students learn theoretically will be practiced and evaluated during practical labs contained within the programs. Sample topics of clinical practice skills for clients of all ages include but are definitely not limited to:

- Assistive technology and devices
- Seating and mobility
- Equipment maintenance
- Splinting/orthotics
- Functional mobility and transfers
- Activities of Daily Living (ADL) training – toileting, bathing, meal preparation, feeding, dressing
- Pediatric interventions
- Fall prevention in multiple environments
- Management of sensory, cognitive, and perceptual dysfunction
- Hand therapy and fine motor skill acquisition
- Mental health interventions
- Occupational participation
- Group interaction skills
- Play and leisure skills
- Care for the older adult

Fieldwork Experience

Clinical education or fieldwork experiences are required for therapist assistant students in both occupational therapy and physiotherapy within the OTA & PTA education accreditation process. Although the number of fieldwork hours does vary across programs, Standard 3.4 of the accreditation standards states that each student must complete a minimum of 500 hours of fieldwork experience in order to graduate. Of the 500 hours, 150 must be in each discipline of occupational therapy and physiotherapy and the remaining 200 hours can be in either, or a combination of occupational therapy and physiotherapy (OTA & PTA EAP, 2018, pp. 28–30). The primary preceptor for each fieldwork placement can be an occupational therapist and/or physiotherapist and/or an OTA/PTA. If the main preceptor is an OTA/PTA, the supervising therapist(s) must be involved in the student evaluation process including signing the evaluation forms. This is a requirement as the OTA/PTA needs therapist supervision while providing client interventions (OTA & PTA EAP, 2014, Guide-06, pp. 2–3).

It can be challenging for therapist assistant education programs to secure OTA student placements – often more difficult than acquiring PTA placements. This problem in locating fieldwork placements is also becoming more difficult for university occupational therapy programs. Alternative opportunities for students to complete fieldwork placement requirements include role-emerging placements and collaborative intraprofessional placements. Both these options will be discussed in further detail.

Role-Established vs. Role-Emerging Placements

It is anticipated that each student will experience fieldwork in a variety of clinical settings with different populations. This will provide a more extensive level of experience upon graduation as an OTA. However, as previously discussed, it can be challenging to secure sufficient placements and clinical preceptors for OTA students as is often similarly the case for student occupational therapists. This has resulted in the development of role-emerging placements.

What is the difference between role-established and role-emerging placements?

- ◆ Role-established fieldwork placements are within clinical settings where roles for the specific discipline, in this context occupational therapy, are established and an occupational therapist is available to clinically supervise the student(s) within the site. Role-established placements will be familiar to education programs, healthcare organizations, and occupational therapists.

◆ Role-emerging fieldwork placements occur within an organization or agency that does not have an established occupational therapy role and supervision is from an off-site occupational therapist (Bossers, Cook, Polatajko, & Laine, 1997, p. 71). For OTA students, a role-emerging placement could also apply to a setting that does have an occupational therapist, but no OTA role has been established.

Role-emerging placements for both occupational therapy students and OTA/PTA students continue to evolve. An example of a role-emerging OTA placement experience within a non-traditional setting occurred at Queen's University within the Continuing Professional Development Office in the Faculty of Health Sciences. As described by Fischer, "as an OTA in this non-traditional setting, I supported an off-site OT in her research and clinical roles" (Fischer & Unsworth, 2016, p. 14), and Fisher's main role in this setting was to "be involved in the qualitative analysis of data obtained through interviews conducted with healthcare professionals who had previously attended continuing medical education programming through the CPD office" (Fischer & Unsworth, 2016, p. 14).

Related to the 2024 Competencies for OTAs, this example would increase the OTA student's skill within Domain F, *Engagement within Occupational Therapy*, as described in the following competency and indicators:

The competent OTA is expected to:

◆ **F3 Contribute to the development of occupational therapy**
  • **F3.1** Help build the occupational therapy body of knowledge.
  • **F3.2** Contribute to research in occupational therapy, innovative practice, and emerging roles of OTAs.
  • **F3.3** Participate in quality improvement initiatives as well as data collection and analysis.

- **F3.4** Collaborate in research with individuals, communities, and people from other disciplines.

(CAOT, 2024b, p. 12)

An example of a role-emerging placement with an occupational therapist on site but no established OTA role was experienced by the same OTA student as in the previous example (Fischer & Unsworth, 2016, p. 14). The OTA student's role in this mental health setting was to "support clients through the leadership and facilitation of occupational therapy activities groups" (Fischer & Unsworth, 2016, p. 15) and "required the application of therapeutic communication strategies in order to support client participation and engagement and to reduce barriers to communication" (Fischer & Unsworth, 2016, p. 15). This experience would increase the student OTA's abilities and confidence within Domain B, *Communication and Collaboration*, of the 2024 Competencies for OTAs, as described below.

The competent OTA is expected to:

- ◆ **B1 Communicate in a respectful and effective manner**
  - **B1.3** Employ communication approaches and technologies suited to the context and client needs (specifically verbal, nonverbal, and written).

(CAOT, 2024b, p. 8)

The occupational therapist preceptor in the latter OTA fieldwork placement example stated that "providing a placement opportunity for an OTA student in a role-emerging fieldwork placement is an excellent way to enhance client care and promote professional learning and development for the OTA student and the practicing/supervising OT" (Fischer & Unsworth, 2016, p. 15). This experience for the preceptor supports Domain F, *Engagement with the Profession*, in the Competencies for occupational therapists, as described below.

The competent occupational therapist is expected to:

◆ **F1 Contribute to the learning of occupational therapists and others**
  - **F1.1** Contribute to entry-to-practice education, such as fieldwork placements.
◆ **F2 Show leadership in the workplace**
  - **F2.1** Support assistants, students, support staff, volunteers, and other team members.
  - **F2.3** Support improvement initiatives at work.
                (ACOTRO, ACOTUP, CAOT, 2021, p. 17)

Students participating in role-emerging placements should be aware of the structure, of how supervision will occur within the placement environment, and that they will need to take initiative, demonstrate motivation, and possibly work independently. This can be challenging for students who may not feel confident in skills such as communication or performing certain treatment techniques, but having completed these role-emerging placements, students often gain valuable experience within their profession in addition to significant personal growth (Bossers, Cook, Polatajko, & Laine, 1997, p. 80).

Clinical fieldwork hours in role-emerging placements *can* be accepted by the OTA & PTA Education Accreditation within the following guidelines:

They make up no more than 150 hours of total placement hours.

◆ They cannot form the only exposure to OTA (or PTA) hours.
◆ An on-site supervisor is available, and this could be a volunteer or a retired occupational therapist who is no longer registered to use title or could be someone with a different background.
◆ An off-site supervisor is available, and this *must* be a registered occupational therapist.
                (OTA & PTA EAP, 2016, Guide-12, pp. 3–4)

Potential sites for OTA role-emerging placements could include the following:

◆ Drop-in centres (pediatric or senior)
◆ Community centres (YMCA)
◆ Group housing programs
◆ Community kitchens for seniors, low-income families
◆ Homeless shelters
◆ Nursery schools
◆ Transition housing settings
◆ Telehealth platforms
◆ Street missions; jails/prisons and halfway release housing
◆ Specific medical vendors
◆ Adapted camps for children

(OTA & PTA EAP, 2016, Guide-12, pp. 4–5)

Activities that OTAs may be providing within these role-emerging placement sites could include:

◆ Being educators re: lifting or transfers for hospitals, vendors
◆ Advisor at airports, hotels, motels for attending to accessibility needs
◆ Inventory and repair, wheelchair cleaning and servicing, cushion sorting at seniors housing that lacks rehab services
◆ Feeding programs
◆ Special projects such as preparing a list of community agencies and providing value-added activities for clients of those agencies.

(OTA & PTA EAP, 2016, Guide-12, p. 5)

Collaboration within Education

Collaboration within healthcare occurs when team members from different professions (interprofessional) and team members from the same profession (intraprofessional) work together to collectively share ideas and create optimal care plans for clients. It is essential that student healthcare workers learn about both interprofessional and intraprofessional collaboration within their education programs.

An intraprofessional fieldwork education study was developed by McMaster University BHSc (OT) Program and Mohawk College OTA/PTA Program in 1997 (Jung, Sainsbury, Grum, Wilkins, & Tryssenaar, 2002). This project explored the collaborative model for student occupational therapists and OTA students learning together during fieldwork placements. Data was collected through journals kept by each student throughout the placement to record "their thoughts, feelings, and concerns arising from their interactions with each other and the preceptors on a regular basis" (Jung, Sainsbury, Grum, Wilkins, & Tryssenaar, 2002, p. 98).

Four common themes emerged from the journals and questionnaires including:

- **Learning about each other's roles**: Many students struggled initially with attempting to understand and accept each other's roles as they related to their own roles. However, most students stated that this improved by the end of the placement.
- **Collaborative learning**: Students understood the importance of collaborative learning although it could be challenging within the team, and sharing a preceptor with another student was difficult at times.
- **Impact on client care and future practice**: Students recognized that an occupational therapist and OTA working together improved the effectiveness and efficiency of occupational therapy services.
- **Resistance to roles**: Some experienced that the supervisory component may have compromised their learning, which was reported by both occupational therapist students and OTA student. This is also indicative of some challenges within real-life practice (Jung, Sainsbury, Grum, Wilkins, & Tryssenaar, 2002, pp. 99–101).

In a further qualitative study by Jung, Salvatori, and Martin in 2008, seven pairs of student occupational therapists and OTA students participated in a unique intraprofessional learning experience that combined a shared fieldwork placement with a small group weekly tutorial. Results indicated that collaborative placements prepare students for clinical practice by:

◆ **Assisting with developing relationships**: The importance of communicating effectively, building trust and respect, and learning together was identified by the participants. An occupational therapist student noted that "the occupational therapist and the OTA need to be on the same page for all clients to be able to chart their progress and report at team meetings" (Jung, Salvatori, & Martin, 2008, p. 46).

◆ **Understanding each other's roles**: This was achieved by the students being informed of defined occupational therapist and OTA roles within the specific environment in addition to role-modeling by those working in the clinical setting. This resulted in improved teamwork.

◆ **Recognizing environmental influences**: Student comments indicated that the collaboration between occupational therapist students and OTA students through tutorials and working within a clinical environment assisted in their learning of the roles and the importance of teamwork. It also provided experience of real-life delivery of healthcare including workload stress and team conflict (Jung, Salvatori, & Martin, 2008, pp. 46–47).

This was reinforced by student occupational therapists from Stanbridge University during a presentation at the 2021 CAOT Virtual Conference. Their poster reviewed a study on assessing therapist/OTA students' perceived readiness to initiate and engage in intraprofessional collaboration. The results indicated that when occupational therapist students and OTA students learn together during their education, they develop a clearer understanding of the occupational therapist and OTA role delineation, standards of practice, and strategies for supervision (Lee, Belk, Engel, Curran, & Scionti, CAOT, 2021). A total of 67 students responded to their survey with the results indicating that: 1. OTA

students were more knowledgeable about supervision requirements than occupational therapy students; 2. Collaboration
improves occupational therapist students and OTA students'
delivery of occupational therapy; and 3. Including this collaboration early in the curriculum better prepares the students to enter
their careers (Lee, Belk, Engel, Curran, & Scionti, CAOT, 2021).

The focus groups conducted by Penner and colleagues in
2020 showed similar concerns with the lack of student collaboration, as evidenced in the second theme they identified as "Living
in the grey, negotiating and navigating the assistant's role". The
study showed that "assistants perceived that they needed to
prove themselves to gain approval and trust, but they also cited
experience as a potential source of conflict when their experience
was substantive, and a therapist was a new graduate" (Penner,
Snively, Packham, Henderson, Principi, & Malstrom, 2020,
p. 401). This is particularly evident if the therapist who recently
graduated had never worked with an OTA during fieldwork.

Another innovative option for fieldwork placements is the
collaborative model of fieldwork education (CMFE). An example
of this model was planned by Murphy & Avvampato in 2021 in
Ontario with an occupational therapy student, two OTA students,
an occupational therapy preceptor (a professor in the OTA/PTA
Diploma program), and an OTA preceptor (an assistant professor
in the MScOT program). The professor preceptors were involved
to "support role clarity and provide structure and support"
(Murphy & Avvampato, 2023, p. 12). As this placement occurred
during COVID-19, they all worked virtually and partnered with
four community organizations to develop resources to support
the occupational therapy needs of each agency (Murphy &
Avvampato, 2023, p. 13). Feedback was provided by the students
throughout the placement and this "OT-OTA CMFE model proved
worthwhile to enable student learners to work together and support community partners" (Murphy & Avvampato, 2023, p. 14).

Interprofessional collaboration, client-centered care, and team
dynamics are necessary skills for all health professionals to learn as
students, including OTAs and PTAs. This concept was integrated
into a hospital setting and involved students from different professions including medicine, nursing, occupational therapy, physiotherapy, and OTA/PTA working together in a clinical environment

(Francis and Strader, 2015, p. 29). An education college where some of the students were enrolled also incorporated an interprofessional introductory course into the healthcare programs to prepare the students to work with other healthcare professionals (Francis and Strader, 2015, p. 29). An OTA and PTA student completed an interprofessional fieldwork placement in the hospital unit under the supervision of both an occupational therapist and a physiotherapist. Interprofessional activities were available for all healthcare students during the placement (Francis and Strader, 2015, p. 29). The OTA and PTA student reported that "through the progression of the placement, my role on the interprofessional team evolved from simple interaction to true collaboration" (Francis and Strader, 2015, p. 30). The course on interprofessional education within the therapist assistant education program also assisted the student to "establish trust with professional colleagues, grounded in a firm understanding of the other professions' scope of practice" (Francis and Strader, 2015, p. 30). This collaborative relationship building between students was a positive experience for the OTA and PTA student, and similarly for the clients based on "positive comments on their [the clients'] level of comfort when working with collaborative teams of students" (Francis and Strader, 2015, p. 30). This type of interprofessional experience would increase the student OTA's abilities and confidence as described within Domain A, *Occupational Therapist Assistant Expertise*, and in Domain B, *Communication and Collaboration* of the 2024 Competencies for OTAs, as described below:

The competent OTA is expected to:

◆ **A4 Perform within the limits of competence within the broad practice context(s)**
  • **A4.2** Seek appropriate consultation from the occupational therapist and other team members.

(CAOT, 2024b, p. 7)

The competent OTA is expected to:

◆ **B1 Communicate in a respectful and effective manner**
  • **B1.5** Recognize and communicate with clients and other professionals the limits of the OTA role.

(CAOT, 2024b, p. 8)

As earlier discussed within this chapter, it is a common challenge for Canadian education programs to secure OTA fieldwork placements. Role-emerging placements and intraprofessional or CMFE placements are alternatives to the role-established placements and need to be incorporated more consistently within the occupational therapist and OTA education programs. The intraprofessional fieldwork placements are often difficult for educational institutions to organize due to scheduling challenges and buy-in from potential preceptors. However, when they have taken place, the results have been very successful. Collaborative occupational therapist and OTA fieldwork placements prepare students for clinical practice by assisting them to develop therapeutic relationships and better understand each other's roles. It also provides opportunities to recognize environmental influences in the delivery of healthcare such as workload stress and team conflict (Jung, Salvatori, & Martin, 2008).

It is imperative to emphasize here that successful fieldwork placements with supportive preceptors for both student occupational therapists and OTA students, or a collaboration of both, will increase each student's confidence as they approach the beginning of their career within the profession of occupational therapy. This is reinforced by the author's experience many years ago but is still extremely effective today. Occupational therapists and OTAs that willingly agree to supervise students in fieldwork placements are participating in their education and preparing them for their careers.

Frequently Asked Questions

1. **Do OTA students learn about Indigenous cultures during their education?**
   It is an expectation that OTA students do learn about Indigenous Peoples in their education programs as this is a recent requirement within occupational therapy practice in Canada.

   As discussed earlier in this chapter, the *Competencies for Occupational Therapist Assistants 2024* contain competencies and indicators for OTAs to demonstrate during their clinical practice, and this requirement will also be updated within the OTA & PTA Education Accreditation Standards. This is reinforced within the *Joint position statement – Toward equity and justice: Enacting an intersectional approach to social accountability in occupational therapy 2024*. The extent to which students learn about Indigenous Peoples within their OTA curriculum will likely vary between education programs and provinces/territories, as well as between accredited and non-accredited education programs. It is beneficial to offer students specific modules on Indigenous Peoples and/or engage with a guest speaker or an educator within the program who has expertise on this topic.

Students' learning about working with Indigenous Peoples also needs to be reinforced by their fieldwork preceptors during clinical placements and needs to be included in the preceptor requirements when preparing to supervise an OTA student within their work setting.

2. **Do OTAs learn how to adjust, maintain, and repair wheelchairs and walkers?**

OTA students learn extensive skills on adjusting, maintaining, and possibly repairing mobility devices including wheelchairs, canes, and walkers – the repairs that are initiated will depend on the extent of what is required. It is also important to note that if a wheelchair is within the warranty period, the vendors need to be contacted for required repairs. These skills are mainly learned through practical lab sessions and may also involve local medical vendors who offer to assist in teaching the OTA students the needed skills.

The extent of each OTA's wheelchair skills will also depend on learning they have acquired within fieldwork placement experiences, additional courses they have completed, and tasks they have been assigned in clinical settings. Additionally, OTAs have recently been more involved in wheelchair seating clinics, an example of a role-emerging position within practice. This could include assisting occupational therapists with wheelchair assessments, completing fitting requirements based on the assigned interventions, connecting and scheduling appointments with medical vendors, and adding extra components to the wheelchair based on the complexity of the parts.

OTAs should be given the responsibility to monitor the condition and safety of the mobility devices owned by clinical settings that are provided to clients on a trial basis until the devices are no longer required or the client receives their permanent device. These settings could include public- or private-funded hospitals, assisted living or long-term care facilities, mental health facilities, community clinics, and home care settings. The overall knowledge and skills of OTAs ensures that devices and equipment within these settings have all the correct components available and are consistently maintained for safe use by the clients within the time frame required.

3. **What occupational therapy treatments do OTA students learn that they could provide to clients?**

This is a common question that is asked during presentations and workshops. There are numerous treatments that OTAs can provide to clients based on their skills and the therapy assignment by the supervising occupational therapist. The five scenarios that follow illustrate potential treatments within certain situations that the author has experienced or learned about in clinical practice and could be included within case studies in an education program.

A. Anna is 72 years of age and lives on the main floor of her daughter's home in a small community. Anna has recently had open heart surgery and reported that her memory had declined since the surgery. She has also reported general weakness resulting in increasing difficulties dressing herself. She was admitted to the local hospital yesterday due to her declined status.

- Anna scored 17/30 on the Saint Louis University Mental Status Exam (or SLUMS) administered by the occupational therapist.
- Two goals agreed to by the occupational therapist and Anna include:
  1. To improve her memory and general cognition
  2. To dress herself independently

With the client's consent, the therapist has decided to assign treatments to the OTA – the therapist and the OTA have worked together for two years.

Treatments that have been assigned by the therapist to the OTA to meet the client's goals include:

Goal #1: To improve her memory and general cognition

- Practice drawing a clock and setting the correct time.
- Match cards with same shapes and colors.
- Play a game that Anna is familiar with, such as cribbage or rummy.

With each of these treatments, the OTA will grade each activity by increasing or decreasing the difficulty based on Anna's cognitive changes.

Goal #2: To dress herself independently

- Visit Anna in her hospital room the first morning and introduce this treatment by the OTA asking Anna to select clothing to wear that day.
- Observe Anna attempt to don lower extremity clothing first and provide recommendations as needed.
- If Anna becomes frustrated or is unable to put on specific clothing, the OTA can provide assistance as appropriate.
- Once the lower limb dressing is completed, the OTA can repeat the same procedure with the upper extremities.

This treatment can be repeated each morning. If Anna is experiencing challenges with independently completing certain activities such as buttoning a shirt or donning supportive footwear, the OTA can introduce the use of assistive devices (buttonhook, elastic shoelaces, long-handled shoehorn).

Following one week of treatment by the OTA, the occupational therapist would determine Anna's progress by completing a reassessment. Anna's treatment program would be adapted based on the evaluation.

B. Harold is 35 years of age and lives with his spouse in a one-level home within the city. They have two children aged eight and five years. Harold experienced severe burns to both hands when gasoline ignited as he was servicing his lawn mower at home. He now has layers of bandages covering his entire hands and wrists.

- Harold shared with the occupational therapist during the assessment that the one occupation he needed to complete independently is feeding himself. He stated he agreed with the nursing staff performing his other care activities, but he did not want them to feed him.

- One initial goal agreed to by the occupational therapist and Harold is:

  1. Independent feeding with use of assistive devices

  Based on this discussion and his main goal of feeding himself independently, the occupational therapist explained to the client that the OTA could fabricate a universal cuff feeding device that could fit around the bandages on his dominant hand and hold a spoon or fork that he could use while eating. This would give him controlled use of the utensils. He agreed to the OTA fabricating this device.

  Goal #1: To feed himself independently

  ■ The occupational therapist assigned to the OTA the task of building a customized universal cuff to fit over the bandages of

Harold's dominant hand that would hold a spoon or a fork to assist with his eating. As the OTA had not fabricated this type of an assistive device recently, the therapist instructed them in the materials to use and showed an example of the finished product —although it was a smaller size to fit over an average hand.

- Once completed, the OTA applied the universal cuff onto Harold's dominant hand and inserted a spoon, and then a fork, explaining the process to use when picking up the food. Harold demonstrated that he could pick up food with the appropriate utensil and feed himself.

- Once the therapist agreed that the cuff was an appropriate fit, the OTA was to educate the nursing staff as to how to apply the universal cuff when Harold's meals were brought to him, and to insert the correct utensil.

The OTA checked with Harold during his meals over the next two days, and evidence indicated the universal cuff was successful. The OTA reported this to the occupational therapist who followed up with a reassessment. Harold informed the therapist that he was pleased he was able to feed himself once fitted with the universal cuff.

C. Mavis is 66 years of age living alone in an apartment with elevator access. They have been diagnosed with osteoarthritis and osteroporosis in addition to sustaining a left shoulder injury approximately one month prior to a referral to community home care. The injury occurred when they attempted to return a heavy frying pan to the bottom drawer of their stove. Mavis is cognitively intact and wants to remain independent in as many personal care activities as possible.

Following the occupational therapist's assessment within Mavis's home environment, two goals that the occupational therapist and Mavis agreed to include:

1. Independence and safety while showering – grab bars had previously been correctly installed
2. Learning joint protection techniques during kitchen tasks

Mavis consents to the OTA to provide treatments within their home environment to assist in meeting these goals. The OTA has worked with the therapist for one year in this community setting.

Treatments provided by the OTA to meet the goals include:

Goal #1: Independence and safety while showering

- The OTA initially observes Mavis transfer into the shower, complete the showering task, and then exit the tub.
- The OTA recommended that Mavis use an assistive device such as a long-handled bath brush and non-slip mats both inside and outside the tub.

Goal #2: Learning joint protection techniques during kitchen tasks

- The OTA made suggestions as to how Mavis could organize their kitchen tools and supplies to decrease the risk of reaching or bending, particularly for heavier pans.
- It was recommended that Mavis use their right arm to protect their left arm from further injury and pain and use larger muscles to support themselves during activities.
- The OTA discussed the option of possibly ordering pre-made meals to be delivered to Mavis's home and they agreed to consider this as an option.

Following the OTA's treatment over three days within a week, the occupational therapist reassessed Mavis's safety during occupational participation in their activities at home. Mavis stated that they were safer within the shower, having purchased non-slip mats, and had less pain performing kitchen tasks. Mavis also decided to initiate a meal program a few days a week.

D. Adam is 18 years of age and has recently been diagnosed with depression following the passing of his father from a motor vehicle accident. Adam has not been participating in activities with his friends including sports and has been hiding himself in his bedroom at home. Adam agreed to attend occupational therapy at a local community centre that focuses on improving occupational participation and social skills of younger adults with mental health symptoms.

Following the occupational therapist's assessment, two goals agreed to by the therapist and Adam are:
1. Improve Adam's social interaction skills
2. Increase Adam's interest in resuming activities with his friends

Adam consents to the OTA providing treatments to work towards meeting these goals. The OTA has been contracted at the community centre for two years and has worked with the occupational therapist throughout that time frame.

Treatments provided by the OTA to meet these goals include:

Goal #1: Improve Adam's social interaction skills
■ Engage Adam in a meaningful activity with the OTA. Initially, the OTA would ask Adam if there is a particular activity, such as a board game, he would like to participate in that is available within the centre. If he does not respond, the OTA would present two activities and have Adam choose one. The OTA would encourage Adam's participation and ask questions during the activity.

- As Adam's participation improved, the OTA would increase the group size to increase social skills development and improve Adam's self-confidence with others through feedback and encouragement throughout the activity. A new activity would be included to increase learning and skill development.

Goal #2: Increase Adam's interest in resuming activities with his friends

- The OTA would initiate conversation with Adam about activities he enjoys with his friends and ask how he feels about resuming these activities.
- Based on Adam's response, the OTA could plan an activity that could slowly increase Adam's confidence in being with others. This could include walking outdoors through the local neighborhood, stopping at a coffee shop, or going to a nearby park. As his confidence increased, the OTA could encourage Adam to reach out to a friend to initiate conversation.
- The OTA would also encourage Adam to journal each day about his successes and limitations.

Following the OTA's treatment with Adam over two weeks, the occupational therapist reassessed Adam. He demonstrated more initiative in participating in activities and stated that he had contacted one of his friends for an initial conversation. He reported that the journaling activity was beneficial in assisting him in reviewing his daily experiences and learning more about his emotions.

E. Klaus is 35 years of age and has recently been diagnosed with carpal tunnel syndrome. He is an agricultural worker on a farm and started noticing tingling and numbness in his dominant right hand mainly in his thumb and index, middle, and ring fingers and was experiencing pain during the night. Klaus was assessed by an occupational therapist in a private practice clinical setting.

Following the assessment, two of the goals recommended by the occupational therapist and agreed to by Klaus are:

1. Reduce Klaus's symptoms of numbness and pain by fabricating a thermoplastic wrist immobilization splint (also referred to as a wrist cockup splint)
2. Regain movement and strength in Klaus's hand and wrist through an exercise program

There is an OTA who works at the clinic who received training about splinting during their therapist assistant education program. The OTA informed the occupational therapist that even though they were guided in fabricating a splint using thermoplastic material during their practical lab session to become familiar working with the material, their instructor reinforced that occupational therapists will be the professionals who fabricate splints in clinical practice work settings.

Klaus agreed to the OTA assisting with the splint fabrication as assigned by the occupational therapist. The roles of an OTA within splint fabrication and completion could include:

◆ Ordering the inventory and maintaining the splinting tools and equipment.
◆ Gathering the required material, tools, and equipment needed for the occupational therapist to fabricate the splint.
◆ Finish the splint by smoothing the surfaces, ensuring there are no sharp edges.
◆ Adding straps onto the splint in the appropriate locations as instructed by the occupational therapist.
◆ Applying the finished splint to the client's limb.
◆ Monitoring the fit of the splint to check for any potential pressure areas.
◆ Adjusting the splint and/or straps as needed.

◆ Teaching wear and care of the splint to the client.
Treatment provided by the OTA to meet the goals
will include:

Goal #1: Reduce Klaus's symptoms of numbness
and pain by the occupational therapist fabricating a thermoplastic wrist immobilization splint
(also referred to as a wrist cockup splint)

- Once the occupational therapist has completed fabricating the splint, the OTA will be
  assigned the finishing of the splint, including
  adding three D-ring pull-through straps in the
  locations indicated by the therapist.
- The OTA will fit the splint onto Klaus and ask
  him if there are any areas of discomfort while
  ensuring the fit of the splint is appropriate and
  safe. The OTA will then make any adjustments
  as needed.
- The OTA will instruct Klaus in how to apply
  the splint, the required tension of the straps,
  when the splint should be worn, as well as any
  precautions/limitations he needs to be aware
  of while wearing the splint and where it is to
  be kept when not in use.
- The OTA will report back to the occupational
  therapist if concerns arise that are out of the
  OTA's responsibilities.
- The OTA will schedule an appointment to
  review the splint in three days.

Goals #2: Regain movement and strength in Klaus's
hand and wrist through an exercise program

- The OTA will instruct Klaus in a hand exercise
  program that has been assigned by the occupational therapist.
- The OTA will use the "tell me, show me,
  watch me do it" teaching approach during the
  instruction.
- Klaus will be asked to complete the exercise program at home within the schedule, frequency,

and repetitions assigned by the occupational therapist.

- The OTA will review Klaus's exercises during the appointment scheduled in three days.

Following the OTA's monitoring of his splint and Klaus performing the hand exercise program, the occupational therapist reassessed Klaus after two weeks. He stated that his pain and numbness were decreased and his hand function had improved.

4. **What form of occupational therapy intervention or treatment principles are taught within the OTA education programs?**

This subject may vary within programs as occupational therapy theory continues to evolve. From the author's perspective as an OTA instructor, a common resource for this topic is the Fundamental Elements of Intervention from the 1991 CAOT *Occupational Therapy Guidelines for Client-Centred Practice*. Although these guidelines are from many years ago, they continue to play a role in OTAs' understanding the principles to apply when providing occupational therapy to clients. The five fundamental elements, or principles, are briefly described below:

◆ **Spirituality**: The centre of a person's being and what brings meaning to their life, including their "spiritual socialization, belief systems and value orientation" (CAOT, 1991, p. 58). A lack of spirituality may appear "through loneliness, depression, sometimes anxiety and feelings of powerlessness" (CAOT, 1991, p. 58).

◆ **Motivation**: Motivation involves thought and emotion, and "is the dynamic or inner force that brings a person to act according to a sense of purpose and direction in life" (CAOT, 1991, p. 59). Clients will be motivated by factors such as their interests and values (spirituality) and the effect of their current illness or disability on their current life roles.

◆ **Therapeutic Relationship**: This is a necessary component in providing treatments to clients and is the topic of Chapter 2. The therapeutic relationship can be seen as a business relationship as an OTA is providing treatments to clients as assigned by the supervising occupational therapist, but it is also "personal and therapeutic although not social or intimate" (CAOT, 1991, p. 61). This means it is more supportive as a client is being treated as a person.

◆ **Teaching Learning Process**: This will assist the client in their development and learning. The learning process "may involve developing problem-solving skills, acquiring new techniques for functioning or gaining new attitudes towards self" (CAOT, 1991, p. 65). One of the principles in this process is "tell me, show me, watch me do it" which was previously discussed in this chapter under Education Trends.

◆ **Ethics**: Ethical dilemmas do occur in occupational therapy practice "considering the pressures for quality assurance and cost control" (CAOT, 1991, p. 66). As stated in Chapter 2 by Corbett, "ethics provide basic principles which individuals within a group can use to determine an appropriate action or response to situations with which they come into contact" (Corbett, 1993, p. 115). A decision-making process by Corbett that results in a morally defensible decision as the outcome is included in Chapter 2 along with situation examples (Corbett, 1993, p. 116).

5. **Do OTA students learn about critical thinking within their education programs?**
Yes, OTA students should learn about critical thinking during their training. They are provided with case studies during course work, assignments, and exams requiring them to use a problem-solving process which is a component of critical thinking. They are taught to analyze information objectively and this often applies to task analysis resulting in grading and/or adapting tasks as needed, based on the client's performance and the limitations documented by the supervising occupational therapist within the supervision plan. This will be discussed in more detail in Chapter 3.

Critical thinking also occurs during fieldwork placements, when OTAs learn how to apply what they have learned theoretically to actual clients in various clinical fieldwork settings through the guidance of their placement preceptor. The preceptor can be an OTA or an occupational therapist, or as described in discussion of role-emerging placements, it could be an off-site occupational therapist. Of note, if the student's preceptor is an OTA, their supervising occupational therapist must also be involved in the student's placement, in particular participating in and signing the student's fieldwork evaluation.

Critical thinking is included the 2024 OTA Competencies within Domain A, *Occupational Therapist Assistant Expertise*:

The competent OTA is expected to:

◆ **A3 Demonstrate effective problem solving and judgment related to assigned service components**
  - **A3.3** Respond to change in status of the client using task analysis and critical thinking.

(CAOT, 2024b, p. 7)

6. **Do student OTAs learn about group facilitation skills?** Group facilitation skills are potentially learned about within their course work and potentially practiced during assignments – for example, asking students to describe a process they might use to teach a group of older adults in a care home a specific activity, and how they would deal with a certain behavioral issue if it occurred during the activity. Practicing group facilitation activities is often experienced during fieldwork placements in a variety of settings. An example of this could be leading a "coffee and conversation" group within a mental health facility to encourage improved social communication skills and ensuring that each group member participates within the activity. Another example is teaching a craft activity within a long-term care facility that each member of the group has expressed an interest in learning.

7. **Can OTAs work in any type of mental health setting?**
   OTAs potentially can work in any mental health setting whether within hospitals, the justice system as inpatients or outpatients, or within community settings. Students learn about mental health during their OTA education, including potential treatments that could be provided through both individual one-on-one sessions and within groups.

   Some examples of mental health settings where OTAs could potentially work under the supervision of an occupational therapist include the following:
   ◆ Working in a homeless shelter where they can teach pertinent life skills to individuals who are transitioning from the shelter into a housing complex. These skills could include self-care, budgeting, grocery shopping, and cooking. In addition, OTAs could assist individuals in participating in other occupations that will allow them to improve their purpose in life as well as supporting them to deal with trauma they may have experienced by becoming homeless. This therapy will provide an overall improvement in the client's well-being.
   ◆ The OTA could assist in teaching a client how to adjust to new social environments and approaches to use in dealing with interpersonal conflict if this has occurred.
   ◆ The OTA could work with clients in a mental health hospital environment who are preparing for discharge home and need to improve their interpersonal communication skills. This would increase their overall confidence in communication but in particular it could also assist them to better participate in job interviews towards potential employment.
   ◆ Within a home care setting, the OTA could teach a client who is afraid to leave their home how to determine the safest and most effective method and route to access required destinations within their community. The type of transportation could include a bus, rail, or ferry service and the OTA could accompany the client through the activity to ensure they understand the process.

◆ OTAs can also work with children who have experienced trauma by assisting with building their self-confidence through activities they enjoy, such as games, dancing, or sports.

References

Association of Canadian Occupational Therapy Regulatory Organizations, Association of Canadian Occupational Therapy University Programs, & Canadian Association of Occupational Therapists. (2021). *Competencies for occupational therapists in Canada.* OT-Competency-Document-EN-HiRes.pdf (acotro-acore.org)

Blake, M., Park, D., & Brice-Leddy, L. (2015). Occupational therapists as practice managers, assistants as primary providers of therapeutic interventions: It's time to talk. *Occupational Therapy Now, 17*(2), 13–15.

Blandford, M. (2018). Occupational therapists and patient flow: Important contributions and opportunities to make a difference. *Occupational Therapy Now, 20*(4), 27–29.

Bossers, A., Cook, J., Polatajko, H., & Laine, C. (1997). Understanding the role-emerging fieldwork placement. *Canadian Journal of Occupational Therapy, 64,* 70–81.

Canadian Association of Occupational Therapists, Association of Canadian Occupational Therapy Regulatory Organizations, & Association of Canadian Occupational Therapy University Programs. (2024). *Joint position statement – Toward equity and justice: Enacting an intersectional approach to social accountability in occupational therapy.* Canadian Association of Occupational Therapists. https://caot.ca/document/8179/Toward%20Equity%20and%20Justice_JPS_EN_V3.pdf

Canadian Association of Occupational Therapists. (2024a). www.caot.ca

Canadian Association of Occupational Therapists. (2024b). *Competencies for occupational therapist assistants.* https://caot.ca/document/8146/Competencies%20OTA%20EN%20Feb%208%202024.pdf

Canadian Association of Occupational Therapists. (1991). *Occupational therapy guidelines for client-centred practice.* Toronto: CAOT Publications ACE.

Canadian Association of Occupational Therapists. (1998). Position statement on support personnel in occupational therapy services. *Canadian Journal of Occupational Therapy, 65*(2), 111–112.

Canadian Occupational Therapist Assistant and Physiotherapist Education Council (COPEC). (2023). http://copec.ca

Canadian Physiotherapy Association. (2024). https://physiotherapy.ca/

Corbett, K. (1993). Ethics and occupational therapy practice. *Canadian Journal of Occupational Therapy, 60*(3), 115–117.

Davidson, K. (2015). Occupational therapist assistants in occupational therapy: An update on the Occupational Therapist Assistant and Physiotherapist Assistant Education Accreditation Program. *Occupational Therapy Now, 17*(2), 11–12.

Douglas, A. (2018). The value of OTA/PTA educational accreditation across Canada. *Occupational Therapy Now, 20*(2), 6.

Egan, M. & Restall, G. (2022). *Promoting occupational participation: Collaborative relationship-focused occupational therapy.* Ottawa: Canadian Association of Occupational Therapists.

Fischer, K. & Unsworth, G. (2016). The development of occupational therapist assistant roles and skillsets through innovative and role-emerging fieldwork opportunities: A student perspective. *Occupational Therapy Now, 18*(6), 14–16.

Francis, D. and Strader, C. (2015). The role of occupational therapist assistant and physiotherapist assistant students on an interprofessional education unit. *Occupational Therapy Now, 17*(2), 29–30.

Gerlach, A. (2012). A critical reflection on the concept of cultural safety. *Canadian Journal of Occupational Therapy, 79*(3), 151–158.

Government of Canada. (2016). *Common definitions on cultural safety: Chief Public Health Officer health professional forum.* https://www.canada.ca/en/health-canada/services/publications/health-system-services/chief-public-health-officer-health-professional-forum-common-definitions-cultural-safety.html

Hagler, P., Madill, H., & Kennedy, L. (1994). Facing choices about our beliefs regarding support personnel. *Canadian Journal of Occupational Therapy, 61*(4), 215–218.

Jung, B., Sainsbury, S., Grum, R.M., Wilkins, S., & Tryssenaar, J. (2002). Collaborative fieldwork education with student occupational therapists and student occupational therapist assistants. *Canadian Journal of Occupational Therapy, 69*(2), 95–103.

Jung, B., Salvatori, P., & Martin, A. (2008). Intraprofessional fieldwork education: Occupational therapy and occupational therapist assistant students learning together. *Canadian Journal of Occupational Therapy*, *75*(1), 42–49.

Lee, A., Belk, A., Engel, C., Curran R., & Scionti, C. (2021). *Poster presentation. Occupational Therapy and Occupational Therapist Assistant Collaboration in Academia. CAOT Virtual 2021 Conference.*

Murphy, S. & Avvampato, T. (2023). Fieldwork collaboration to overcome system-level challenges. *Occupational Therapy Now*, *26*(3), 12–14.

Occupational Therapist Assistant and Physiotherapist Assistant Education Accreditation. (2013). https://www.otapta.ca/english/index.php

Occupational Therapist Assistant and Physiotherapist Assistant Education Accreditation Program. (2014). *Guide-06 supervision of OTA/PTA students during fieldwork.* https://otapta.ca/pdfs/About%20Us/FAQs/GUIDE-06%20Supervision%20of%20OTA%20PTA%20Students%20During%20Fieldwork.pdf

Occupational Therapist Assistant and Physiotherapist Assistant Education Accreditation Program. (2016). *Policy & procedures GUIDE-12 role emerging clinical placements, Mar 2016.* https://otapta.ca/pdfs/About%20Us/FAQs/GUIDE-12%20Role%20Emerging%20Placements.pdf

Occupational Therapist Assistant and Physiotherapist Assistant Education Accreditation Program. (2018). *Accreditation standards.* 2012 OTA PTA EAP Accreditation Standards - 2018 Revision FINAL.pdf

Occupational Therapist Assistant and Physiotherapist Assistant Education Accreditation Program. (2020). *Program accreditation handbook.* OTAPTA EAP Program Handbook (current).pdf

Penner, J.D., Snively, A., Packham, T.L., Henderson, J., Principi, E. & Malstrom, B. (2020). Viewpoints of the occupational therapist assistant – Physiotherapy assistant role on inter-professional teams: A mixed-methods study. *Physiotherapy Canada*, *72*(4). https://doi.org/10.3138/ptc-2019-0011

Salvatori, P. (2001). The history of occupational therapy assistants in Canada: A comparison with the United States. *Canadian Journal of Occupational Therapy*, *68*(4), 217–227.

Vo, L. & Feenstra, C. (2015). The emerging role of occupational theorist assistants at The Ottawa Hospital. *Occupational Therapy Now*, *17*(2), 23.

von Zweck, C. & Gillespie, H. (1998). Support personnel in occupational therapy: Who, what, why and how. *Canadian Journal of Occupational Therapy*, *65*(2), 59–63.

World Federation of Occupational Therapists. (2019). *Position statement: Occupational therapy and rehabilitation.* https://wfot.org/resources/occupational-therapy-and-rehabilitation

World Federation of Occupational Therapists. (2022). *Guiding principles for competency in occupational therapy.* https://wfot.org/resources/guiding-principles-for-competency-in-occupational-therapy

2

Developing Trusting Relationships

Objectives

After completing this chapter, the reader will be able to:

- ♦ Apply strategies to develop and implement effective occupational therapist/OTA working relationships.
- ♦ Recognize factors that may affect this intraprofessional partnership in addition to interprofessional relationships.
- ♦ Understand the importance of communication within working relationships.
- ♦ Be aware of ethical considerations and how to respond in an ethical dilemma.
- ♦ Understand the occupational therapist/OTA relationship from an OTA perspective.

Key Terms

- ♦ Intraprofessional relationship
- ♦ Interprofessional collaboration
- ♦ Psychosocial safety

DOI: 10.4324/9781003498391-2

◆ Therapeutic relationship
◆ Communication
◆ Ethics

Frequently Asked Questions (FAQs) are included at the end of this chapter.

Intraprofessional Relationship

Prior to addressing the task assignment process, it is necessary to highlight the importance of developing a trusting, working relationship between occupational therapists and OTAs. This relationship includes "good communication skills and a comprehensive understanding of each other's roles and responsibilities" (Stephenson, 2015, p. 28). McCready-Wirth and colleagues further reinforce that "mutual trust needs to be built between the therapist and assistant for effective and efficient service delivery" (McCready-Wirth, Hepting, Ng, Haney, Bratkoski, & MacAusland-Berg, 2015, p.19). This is a necessity particularly in more remote environments such as community and home care settings.

Collaborative relationship-focused approaches for both occupational therapists and OTAs assist in the exploration of the meaning and purpose of occupation (CAOT, 2024, p. 2).

As previously discussed, the *Competencies for Occupational Therapists in Canada (COTC)* 2021 states within Domain A, *Occupational Therapy Expertise*, that:

The competent occupational therapist is expected to:

◆ **A7 Manage the assignment of services to assistants and others**
  • **A7.1** Identify practice situations where clients may benefit from services assigned to assistants or others.
  • **A7.2** Assign services only to assistants and others who are competent to deliver the services.

- **A7.3** Monitor the safety and effectiveness of assignments through supervision, mentoring, teaching, and coaching.
- **A7.4** Follow the regulatory guidance for assigning and supervising services.

(ACOTRO, ACOTUP, CAOT, 2021, p. 11)

This competency and the related indicators demonstrate the importance of developing trusting relationships between occupational therapists and OTAs to enable the occupational therapist to manage the assignment of services effectively and safely to OTAs.

This is reiterated in the CAOT *Competencies for Occupational Therapist Assistants* within Domain A, *Occupational Therapist Assistant Expertise*:

The competent OTA is expected to:

◆ **A1 Establish trusted professional relationships with supervising occupational therapist(s) and clients**
- **A1.1** Co-create with occupational therapist(s) a shared understanding of their roles and expectations.
- **A1.2** Adhere to occupational therapist regulation pertinent to task *assignment* and *supervision*.
- **A1.3** Demonstrate an understanding of *occupational participation*.
- **A1.4** Respond to client assignments, requesting clarification when required.
- **A1.5** Inform clients that OTAs work under the direction and supervision of the occupational therapist.

(CAOT, 2024, p. 7)

This competency and indicators reinforce the requirement for both occupational therapists and OTAs to understand the process of developing a trusting and professional relationship.

The outcome of building a trusting relationship empowers an OTA to say to the assigning therapist "I don't feel comfortable with this intervention – can you review the best process I should

use to instruct the client?" or "I'm experiencing challenges working with this client – can you guide me in the best way to deal
with these issues?" In addition, a trusting relationship enables
the therapist to give more responsibility to the OTA, with confidence increasing in the OTA's competence as the relationship
develops. The occupational therapist is also more comfortable
providing feedback to the OTA as needed to improve occupational therapy service delivery.

The importance of communication in building positive occupational therapist and OTA relationships is reinforced through the
results from Stephenson's qualitative research study. It describes
four types of communication that are valuable to incorporate:

- ◆ Patient-specific communication that relates to treatment assignments, safety, and client updates.
- ◆ Work-related communication describes scheduling,
  indirect activities, and organizational tasks.
- ◆ Peer-based communication in interactions with the
  interprofessional team.
- ◆ Personal communication is sharing information on
  specific interests and personal situations including
  health or family.

(Stephenson, 2015, p. 28)

However, there is evidence in the literature that effective communication and therapists' confidence in working with assistants is not consistent in occupational therapy service delivery,
resulting in less involvement of OTAs in providing treatments.

A recently published international scoping review of the
deployment of Support Workers and Assistant Practitioners
(SWAP), including OTAs within Allied Health Professions (AHP)
involving occupational therapy, reported that the reluctance of
therapists to delegate (or *assign*, the term currently recommended
in Canada) is a factor impeding the effective utilization of this
workforce. However, this often depends on the "level of trust
between the registered professional and the SWAP. Delegation
appears to increase over time, suggesting that once trust had
been developed and competence demonstrated, AHPs were more

comfortable with delegating more highly skilled work to SWAPs" (Etty, Snaith, Hinchcliffe, & Nightingale, 2024, p. 2264).

The factors referenced within Canadian literature include:

1. **Misunderstandings by managers, leadership, and organization of OTA education and their role within therapy delivery**

   Findings from a qualitative research study by Stevenson (2015) and a mixed-methods study design including surveys followed by focus groups by Penner et al. (2020) indicate that there are frequent misunderstandings by managers, leadership, and organizations regarding the education received by OTAs who have graduated from an accredited diploma program, and their role in the delivery of therapy.

   As was discussed in Chapter 1, Hagler, Madill, and Kennedy stated in response to CAOT's affirmation of the section of the 1993 report by Hagler and colleagues at the University of Alberta that support personnel need to be supervised by occupational therapists, and that it is also "incumbent upon the employers, clinical administrators, programme supervisors, clinical professionals, and support workers themselves to ensure that support workers do not provide occupational therapy services without supervision by an occupational therapist" (Hagler, Madill, & Kennedy, 1994, p. 216). As the education and roles of therapist assistants are continuing to evolve, this is an ongoing requirement. This is even more of an issue currently as many managers and leaders do not have a clear understanding of the occupational therapy profession in general.

2. **Therapists' lack of training in the principles of supervision of therapist assistants**

   This is evident through semi-structured interviews discussed during a poster presentation at the 2018 CAOT Conference (Donnellan & Gerlach, CAOT Conference, 2018), and the mixed-methods research study by

Penner, Snively, Packham, Henderson, Principi, & Malstrom (2020).

As reviewed in Chapter 1, these studies reinforce the need for occupational therapists to learn in their university education about their responsibilities for assigning to and supervising OTAs which is enhanced through initially developing a trusting working relationship potentially through intraprofessional student fieldwork placements.

As the OTA role evolves, there also needs to be ongoing professional development education on this topic for occupational therapists and OTAs.

3. **Therapists' discomfort in providing feedback to OTAs**

This was another factor affecting the occupational therapist and OTA relationship, as described by Penner et al. (2020), and relates back to the essential need of investing time to develop a trusting working relationship between therapists and assistants.

(Penner, Snively, Packham, Henderson, Principi, & Malstrom, 2020, p. 401)

An additional subject that needs to be understood by everyone involved in a client's care plan in which the OTA performs interventions assigned to them by the supervising occupational therapist(s) is the format and frequency that has been established in the documented supervision plan (discussed in more detail in Chapter 3). If two occupational therapists job share, and both have assigned interventions to the OTA, the supervisor would be the occupational therapist working that day. In this situation, it is beneficial if both occupational therapists can agree on the tasks assigned and the reporting frequency and structure in order to provide both the OTAs and the clients with a more seamless treatment plan.

This collaboration also needs to be clearly understood by employers, site managers, and interprofessional team members. It is becoming increasingly evident that managers and practice leaders within certain work organizations are pressuring occupational therapists to assign tasks to OTAs that either are inappropriate or create supervision challenges for the therapist, resulting in a safety risk for the clients. Further education must be provided at all levels of management to ensure the overall understanding of the occupational therapist's accountability and supervision requirements for delivery of therapy services that are assigned to OTAs.

Interprofessional Collaboration

It is necessary to discuss therapist assistant roles and limitations within the interprofessional healthcare team and to collaborate as a team to provide optimal care to the clients. Following up on Francis and Strader's description of students experiencing placements on an Interprofessional Education (IPE) Unit within a hospital setting (as discussed in Chapter 1), the opportunity to learn about interprofessional collaboration within OTA & PTA education programs would "provide students with the foundational knowledge and skills necessary to demonstrate optimal interprofessional competence" (Francis & Strader, 2015, p. 30).

It is common practice that OTA/PTAs are assigned both occupational therapy and physical therapy to the same client/patient. In these circumstances, it must be made clear to the OTA/PTA which aspect of the treatment is occupational therapy and which is physical therapy. This clarification will ensure that the correct supervisor is contacted if a question or issue arises during treatment. Whether specific aspects of the assigned treatment are physiotherapy or occupational therapy cannot be assumed based on each profession's "scope of practice," as the definition of "scope" is usually quite broad.

A collaborative interprofessional relationship between occupational therapists and physiotherapists and the OTA(s)/PTA(s) is required to ensure safe and effective therapy provision resulting in the best outcomes for patients/clients. However, this does not always occur in clinical practice, as is evident from the mixed-methods study by Penner and colleagues, within *Theme 3: Who's the Boss?*. Evidence from the study indicated that therapist assistants often experience "conflicting priorities for demands on their time when this time was shared between occupational therapy and physiotherapy" (Penner, Snively, Packham, Henderson, Principi, & Malstrom, 2020, p. 401).

An example of a successful interprofessional collaboration within a community home care environment from the author's experience will now be shared. The OTA/PTA on the team provided client treatments assigned by the occupational therapist and treatments assigned by the physiotherapist. The assistant demonstrated a clear understanding as to which treatments were physiotherapy, and which were occupational therapy, and therefore which supervising therapist to report to if an issue occurred. While planning their schedule on a particular day, the occupational therapist became aware of an unexpected situation with a client that was shared by another team member. Based on the circumstances involved, the occupational therapist asked the OTA/PTA if they could visit this client during a certain time frame later in the day rather than keeping their planned visit on the following day. The OTA/PTA responded that they were already scheduled to see a client for physiotherapy treatment at that time. The occupational therapist then initiated discussion concerning this situation with the supervising physiotherapist, making it clear that if the assigned physiotherapy treatment needed to be delivered as planned, the occupational therapist could adjust their plans and visit the client themselves. Following the communication, the physiotherapist agreed that the occupational therapy client treatment needed to take priority based on the unexpected situation and informed the OTA/PTA that the physiotherapy appointment could be rescheduled for the next day. This example demonstrates that in certain situations the supervising therapists need to initiate communications with the interprofessional team to ensure the best client outcomes, as well as demonstrating the importance of interprofessional collaborations.

Within an acute care hospital setting, the need for clients to be discharged as soon as they are determined to be safe and able to return to their home or other living situation is becoming more of a priority because of the increasing challenges in healthcare environments. An example of how an interprofessional collaboration could promote timely discharges will be discussed. An older client has experienced a fall on the icy sidewalk outside their home which resulted in a lower back injury. The pain is preventing them from dressing their lower extremities themselves and ambulating independently. As the pain decreases, the physiotherapist assigns mobilization practice using a two-wheeled walker and the occupational therapist assigns lower extremity dressing practice to the same OTA/PTA who works on the unit. Due to their heavy workloads and the desire for the client to return home as soon as possible, the therapists and the OTA/PTA meet to briefly discuss how to coordinate these two treatments to ensure that they are delivered in a timely yet safe and effective manner. The team agrees that the OTA/PTA will visit the client in their hospital room following breakfast each morning to practice dressing their lower limbs and to teach the use of assistive devices as needed. Once this activity is completed, and based on the client's physical status and comfort level, the OTA/PTA can then set up the two-wheeled walker and teach the client to safely walk with the support of the walker, initially walking a short distance and returning to their room. The distance walked would be graded up each day based on the client's progress. The OTA/PTA could also return to see the client later each day to ambulate again if the OTA/PTA determined this would be best for the client. The OTA/PTA would document each session and report to each therapist as to the client's progress and any issues that arose. This interprofessional collaboration will provide the client with their required occupational therapy and physiotherapy on a timely basis, with each team member agreeing to this approach.

The importance of interprofessional collaboration is further reinforced in the following example. A team member from another discipline who is working with the same client as the OTA asks the OTA to perform the assigned occupational therapy task in a different way for a particular reason. In this situation, the OTA needs to state that the supervising occupational therapist must be involved in this discussion and make the appropriate decision. If the request is related to a safety concern observed by the other healthcare professional, it is recommended that the

OTA stop the treatment and follow up with the occupational therapist to ensure the client's safety. The therapist would then collaborate with the healthcare professional to create a new plan as needed.

It also needs to be clearly understood by the occupational therapist, the OTA, and interprofessional team that if the OTA is asked to perform a different treatment for a client to whom they are already delivering an assigned occupational therapy treatment, the supervisor for this new treatment is the person who assigned the treatment to the OTA. This could be a physiotherapist, a nurse, a speech language pathologist, or another member of the team, but the supervisor would not be the occupational therapist as they have not assigned this new treatment. This brings up the question as to whether OTA/PTAs should be assigned tasks by nurses. Penner and colleagues also reinforce this question by describing the "difficulty of balancing the demands from rehabilitation versus assisting with nursing care duties delegated by the nursing manager" (Penner, Snively, Packham, Henderson, Principi, & Malstrom, 2020, p. 401).

This is an issue that occurs frequently and definitely needs to be discussed within the interprofessional team. If a nurse asks an OTA/PTA to perform a task with a patient, the nurse is responsible for the supervision and the overall safety of the patient.

It is imperative that all healthcare settings including hospitals, community agencies, school settings, privately funded clinics, long-term care facilities, and mental health services provide psychosocial safety within their environments for all workers, including occupational therapists and OTAs. This will minimize psychosocial hazards such as bullying and disrespect within the workplace which results in stress and potential interpersonal challenges for those staff members affected. OTAs have communicated that there often is a strong dynamic in various work environments across the country where they feel humiliated and disrespected by therapists, leaders and/or managers, and also by other co-workers. Each member of a healthcare team, including occupational therapists and OTAs, must feel supported and confident communicating with each other in their workplace. In addition, the therapists and assistants must also demonstrate responsibility through contributing to the development of workplace cultures that are psychosocially safer, with an emphasis on creating a welcoming environment for recently hired colleagues.

Developing the Occupational Therapist and OTA Therapeutic Relationship

It is mainly the occupational therapist's responsibility to ensure that sufficient time is taken to develop this relationship along with the manager/employer's support. The OTA does have responsibility in building the relationship, but due to the occupational therapist being accountable for client safety and outcomes, this relationship should be initiated by the therapist.

The process described below is one that was developed by the author based on extensive intraprofessional experiences working as an occupational therapist. This process has been used as a mentoring tool for occupational therapists and physiotherapists, as well as student occupational therapists and physiotherapists who have not yet had experience working with therapist assistants.

The first step in the process is that the occupational therapist and the OTAs take the time to become more familiar with each other.

The supervising occupational therapist will initiate and support the professional relationship by:

◆ Sharing past work involvement with OTAs and their experience in the current work setting.
◆ Discussing general expectations of an OTA including communication and responsibilities, in addition to reviewing the pertinent Regulatory College practice guideline/standard related to occupational therapy assignment to OTAs and supervision requirements.
◆ Obtaining informed consent from the client or substitute decision maker (SDM) to have the OTA present during a new client assessment or a client reassessment, if there is the strong potential that the OTA will be involved in

the client's treatment plan. This assists the OTA in understanding the occupational therapist's approach to client care at the beginning of their working relationship.

◆ Providing ongoing supervision and support as needed for assigned treatments.
◆ Sharing personal communication strengths and weaknesses.

The occupational therapist's understanding about OTA colleagues can be achieved by asking the following questions:

◆ The OTA's education related to occupational therapy – did they graduate from an OTA/PTA accredited diploma program?
◆ What has been their previous work experience as an OTA and/or PTA, or in other similar roles?
◆ What types of supervision did they experience within previous work environments (direct, indirect, remote)?
◆ What is their experience with legal documentation/ charting?
◆ Do they have any special interests that could apply to this role?
◆ What are their personal communication strengths and weaknesses?

Since any therapeutic relationship will also involve the client, it is also the occupational therapist's responsibility to ensure the client's safety and transparency by:

◆ Confirming that the client and family members understand the roles and responsibilities of the OTA, including working under the direction/supervision of the occupational therapist.
◆ Obtaining informed consent from the client or substitute decision maker (SDM) for involvement of the OTA in the assigned tasks/interventions.
◆ Reinforcing to the OTA the need to confirm informed consent for initial and ongoing service provision.

> ◆ Ensuring the client understands that anything they discuss with the OTA and/or that the OTA witnesses must be reported back to the occupational therapist (Gillespie, 2023, p. 11).

It is necessary to reinforce that OTAs must be aware of their responsibilities and limits of competence while providing occupational therapy treatments and that safety for both the client and themselves is taken into account at all times. This is contained within the CAOT *Competencies for Occupational Therapist Assistants* within Domain A, *Occupational Therapist Assistant Expertise*:

> **The competent OTA is expected to:**
>
> ◆ **A3 Demonstrate effective problem solving related to assigned service components**
>   - **A3.1** Apply relevant and current occupational therapy knowledge to the practice area.
>   - **A3.2** Ensure client and personal safety in the performance of assigned components of service delivery.
>   - **A3.3** Respond to change in status of the client using task analysis and critical thinking.
> ◆ **A4 Perform within the limits of competence within the broad practice context(s)**
>
>   - **A4.1** Recognize and communicate the limits of individual competence and role.
>   - **A4.2** Seek appropriate consultation from the occupational therapist and team members.
>
> (CAOT, 2024, p. 7)

Clients can often be treated by OTAs more frequently than they are by occupational therapists in many clinical settings, resulting in the development of stronger and more comfortable therapeutic relationships. There also may be a "decreased perceived authority differential between the client and the OTA compared to the client and the occupational therapist" (Gillespie & Engel, 2015, p. 9). This means the client is aware that the occupational therapist has overall responsibility for the therapy provided by the OTA, as well as potentially requesting funding from a third-party funder for assistive devices, environmental adaptations, or other resources. They may not be comfortable expressing any concerns or emotions directly to the occupational therapist, but may often feel safer expressing their feelings to the OTA. Examples of this could include:

- ◆ The OTA is practicing bathtub transfers with the client, using a tub transfer bench in their home. At the end of the practice, the client says, "My wife does not want me to use this bench as it makes me look old and disabled." The OTA would respond by saying something like "I hear your concerns, and I will pass this on to the occupational therapist." The client would then likely say, "That's OK, I just was not comfortable about telling the therapist myself."
- ◆ The OTA is instructing the client in cognitive retraining activities. The client suddenly becomes upset and says to the OTA, "I am really scared that I might have to go into one of those nursing home places because I can't remember anything anymore." The OTA would respond on the lines of "I understand what you're saying and I will let the occupational therapist know your concerns." To this the client might well say, "OK, I was just too scared to say this to anyone else."

It is imperative that supervising therapists and OTAs ensure the clients understand that information, certain questions, or emotional responses shared with the OTA will need to be forwarded to the supervising occupational therapist as they are accountable for the clients' overall therapy delivery and outcomes.

Effective Communication

As already discussed, effective communication is critical in developing successful occupational therapist and OTA relationships. In her book *Emotional Magnetism: How to Communicate to Ignite Connection in Your Relationships*, Sandy Gerber states that

"To engage someone, you need to communicate with them in such a way that they become enthusiastic about what you are saying" (Gerber, 2022, p. 15). This resource provides insight into the development of both intraprofessional and interprofessional working relationships.

Gerber describes three things that work together to create positive relationships:

1. **Empathy** – your ability to understand where a person is coming from. You need to demonstrate that you care about their situation even though you may not agree with what they are communicating.
2. **Authenticity** – your ability to know yourself and understand how you impact others through your actions and words.
3. **Positive regard of others** – your ability to take others' situations seriously leading to them feeling respected.

Applying empathy, authenticity, and positive regard within your relationships, you are able to understand the other person, and you will also be better understood.
(Adapted with permission from S. Gerber (2022),
*Emotional Magnetism: How to Communicate
to Ignite Connection in your Relationships*,
NEXT IMPACT Press, pp. 25–26)

Based on the title of the book, Gerber describes people's emotional needs that impact relationships, calling them Emotional Magnets. They fall into four categories:

- ◆ Safety
- ◆ Achievement
- ◆ Value
- ◆ Experience

The acronym **S.A.V.E.** is a way to remember these four Emotional Magnets.

(Gerber, 2022, p.17)

Those who are magnetized by each of these emotional needs could include people who:

Safety

1. Plan their day and need to know what happens next – attempt to avoid spontaneity.
2. Help others to prepare for life, learn skills, or stay healthy.
3. Want to gain proficiency in new skills.
4. Minimize risk as much as possible.

Achievement

1. Consistently are driven to meet their goals.
2. Enjoy being recognized as a topic expert in their area of expertise.
3. Are dedicated to their career.
4. Enjoy paying it forward through mentoring or coaching.

Value

1. Appreciate receiving recognition from the boss for a specific activity or initiative.
2. Provide growth for themselves and others.
3. Ensure resources are not wasted.
4. Engage in activities that have significance to others.

Experience

1. Are eager and curious to learn new skills.
2. Adapt an activity to make it more enjoyable for themselves and/or others.
3. Enjoy meeting new people.
4. Are motivated by spontaneity and change – may take on too much.

> (Adapted with permission from Gerber, 2022, pp. 54, 55, 60, 69, 72, 85, 88, 89, 96, 98, and 99)

Sandy Gerber's book also includes a quiz that assists readers to determine their own strongest Emotional Magnets (Gerber, 2022, pp. 111–121).

An example is provided below on how these Emotional Magnets can potentially be incorporated into the development of an effective occupational therapist/OTA relationship.

Emotional Magnets: Case Example

The occupational therapist is accountable for safe and effective occupational therapy provided to their clients. This includes being responsible for delivery of treatments they have assigned to an OTA.

If the occupational therapist's main emotional magnet is Safety and the OTA's main emotional magnet is Experience, how would the development of the occupational therapist/OTA working relationship be most successful?

The occupational therapist needs to ensure that the established goals agreed to by the clients are the focus of the therapy but also that potential risks during treatment are identified and minimized as much as possible. Those drawn to Safety also want to be in control as much as possible. This could create a challenge when deciding to assign a client treatment to an OTA, particularly if the treatment is to be delivered in an environment where the therapist cannot provide direct supervision, such as in the client's home.

The OTA's role is delivering occupational therapy treatments as assigned by the supervising occupational therapist to assist clients' in meeting their goals while ensuring the safety of everyone involved. When the OTA's main emotional magnet is Experience, they want to be creative in the treatment provided and have the client progress to their goals in a timely manner. OTAs often tend to develop strong therapeutic relationships with clients as they work with them more frequently, and getting to know people is a strength of those who are Experience oriented.

What is the most effective way to ensure that appropriate communication is used to develop this occupational therapist/OTA relationship in addition to the occupational therapist/OTA/client relationship?

Both the occupational therapist and the OTA need to be aware of the importance of effective communication to ensure quality of care and safety for the involved clients.

As explained earlier in this chapter, the occupational therapist would initiate the conversation to develop the intraprofessional relationship by introducing themselves to the OTA, including their personal communication strengths and weaknesses. The therapist would then ask the OTA to share information about themselves and the ways they view their communication.

The therapist will inform the OTA that the client's goals will be shared with the OTA once client consent for OTA involvement has been given. Potential risks will also be reviewed with the OTA and ways they can be mitigated during treatment. The pertinent occupational therapy regulatory document should be reviewed with the OTA to ensure the OTA's understanding of both the therapist and their own responsibilities.

Based on this example with the therapist's main emotional magnet being Safety, the occupational therapist will inform the OTA of the importance of communicating with the therapist regarding questions, concerns, and clients' progress. The preferred methods of communication will also be reinforced.

As the OTA's main emotional magnet is Experience, they need to understand that if they have a creative idea of a different treatment they have previously used with clients or potential ways to adapt treatments, they need to discuss this with the occupational therapist to ensure the therapist agrees. As the occupational therapist/OTA relationship develops and trust is built, the therapist may give the OTA greater boundaries in adapting the treatments, but initially within the relationship, this important communication needs to occur. The OTA also needs to be aware of their client schedule and to communicate with their supervising therapists if they are unable to take on new clients due to a full schedule. If a supervising therapist wanted to assign a new client treatment, this could be exciting for the OTA drawn to Experience as it is the opportunity to learn a new skill. However, they need to be aware that they can only work with a certain number of clients throughout the day.

When you understand your own and others' Emotional Magnets, communication is more empathetic, resulting in minimizing misunderstandings and developing more effective working relationships.

Ethics

What do we mean by *ethics* and what could the impact be in both intraprofessional and interprofessional relationships? The World Federation of Occupational Therapists' recent 2024 document *Guiding Principles for Ethical Occupational Therapy* states that "occupational therapists must be accountable to society for the use of their expertise in the service of others. Being accountable requires that the principles, values, and beliefs that guide work in occupational therapy are clear for members of the profession, individuals receiving occupational therapy and others" (WFOT, 2024, p. 1). This applies to OTAs who are members of the profession and provide occupational therapy treatments under the supervision of occupational therapists. WFOT describes ten occupational values and beliefs that apply to ethical occupational therapy practice. These include:

1. **Occupation focus**: "Occupational therapists work with individuals, groups and communities in a variety of settings to promote participation in occupations that give value and meaning to life" (WFOT, 2024, p. 3). This would also apply to OTAs working under the supervision of occupational therapists.

2. **Collaborative Approach**: "Occupational therapy uses a holistic perspective, recognizing the biological, psychological, social, cultural and spiritual dimensions of individuals, groups and communities that access services" (WFOT, 2024, p. 4).

3. **Duty of Care**: "The primary professional responsibility of occupational therapists is to people receiving occupational therapy, whether individuals, families, communities or populations. They have a duty to avoid injury, loss or damage as a result of their actions, and to diligently respond to incidents" (WFOT, 2024, p. 4). This includes matters of ethical concern.

4. **Human rights and occupational justice**: "Occupational therapists recognize that health is a human right and incorporate justice, transparency and accountability in

their practice" (WFOT, 2024, p. 4). This includes collaborations with OTAs.

5. **Respect for diversity**: Those working in occupational therapy "consider the cultural diversity, lifestyles and perspectives of the people they serve and do not discriminate on the basis of race, ability, national origin, age, gender, sexual preference, religion, political beliefs or status in society" (WFOT, 2024, p. 4).

6. **Integrity**: "Occupational therapists maintain standards of conduct at all times and demonstrate personal integrity, honesty, reliability, open-mindedness and loyalty. They serve in the best interest of the public, guided by a defined set of competencies, standards and ethics, and aligned with laws, regulations and policies within the circumstances in which services are provided" (WFOT, 2024, p. 5).

7. **Confidentiality**: "Occupational therapists respect the right of all individuals for confidentiality and privacy" (WFOT, 2024, p. 5).

8. **Competency and life-long learning:** "Occupational therapists are autonomous professionals who make individual judgments in the provision of services for which they have knowledge, skills and abilities" (WFOT, 2024, p. 5).

9. **Obligations to the profession**: "The occupational therapy profession formulates standards of practice and conduct that adhere to ethical values, attitudes and behaviours to enable self-regulation" (WFOT, 2024, p. 6).

10. **Responsibility toward local and global societies**: "Occupational therapy spans multiple sectors beyond health, including education, labour, and social development. In all areas, occupational therapy has an obligation to promote the use of resources to deliver services in a way that does not compromise the health of present or future generations" (WFOT, 2024, p. 6).

These guiding principles need to be consistently incorporated into intraprofessional occupational therapy service delivery when occupational therapists have assigned treatments to OTAs to ensure that all clients receive safe, effective, and ethical occupational therapy.

What is meant by the term "ethics"? Corbett states that "ethics provide basic principles which individuals within a group can use to determine an appropriate action or response to situations with which they come into contact" (Corbett, 1993, p. 115). Therefore, occupational therapists and OTAs need to demonstrate ethical competence throughout their careers.

The Canadian Association of Occupational Therapists Code of Ethics (2018) describes the ethical expectations of its members. It states that occupational therapists must follow their regulatory organization's Code of Ethics requirements which include that the OTAs they are supervising are also aware of ethical expectations during provision of occupational therapy treatments.

The *Competencies for Occupational Therapists in Canada 2021* includes within Domain E, *Professional Responsibility*, the following competency and indicators:

The competent occupational therapist is expected to:

◆ **E1 Meet legislative and regulatory requirements**
- **E1.1** Respect the laws, codes of ethics, rules and regulations that govern occupational therapy.
- **E1.5** Respond to ethical dilemmas based on ethical frameworks and client values.
- **E1.8** When observed, respond to and report unprofessional, unethical, or oppressive behaviour, as required.
    (ACOTRO, ACOTUP, & CAOT, 2021, p. 16)

The *Competencies for Occupational Therapist Assistants (2024)* document also includes these ethical requirements within Domain E, *Professional Responsibility*:

The competent OTA is expected to:

◆ **E1 Work within the legislative and regulatory requirements for occupational therapists**
- **E1.1** Respect the laws, codes of ethics, rules, and regulations that govern occupational therapy.

- **E1.5** Respond to ethical dilemmas based on ethical frameworks and client values.
- **E1.8** Respond to and report observed unprofessional, unethical, or oppressive behaviour, as required.

(CAOT, 2024, p. 11)

Examples of ethical dilemma scenarios that involve an OTA could include:

1. An occupational therapist in a rural community has assessed a client following a motor vehicle accident. The occupational therapist has assigned an exercise program to the OTA who has recently moved back to this community. While reviewing the assignment, the OTA realizes that this client was a classmate ten years ago, and they have mutual friends. What does the OTA do?

2. A team colleague in a return-to-work clinical setting makes a racist comment in the staff room about an Indigenous client whom the OTA is also treating. The client experienced a shoulder dislocation following a work injury as a heavy-duty mechanic and is anxious to return to their job as soon as possible. What does the OTA do?

3. An OTA is contracted at a complex care facility in a full-time position. The supervising occupational therapist is at the facility two days/week. The nurse approaches the OTA stating that the status of the resident in room 101 has declined over the past two days. The nurse then requests that the OTA contact the resident's daughter who is very involved in their mother's care. The daughter can then guide the OTA in any changes that need to be made to the occupational therapy treatment plan. How does the OTA respond?

4. The OTA has been treating a client following a back injury, and the occupational therapist is planning a reassessment to determine potential discharge by the end of the week. The client works as an accountant and has kindly offered to complete the OTA's tax return at a reduced cost.

The deadline for filing the return is fast approaching and the OTA has not yet finished this task. How should the OTA respond?

5. An OTA has been treating a client daily in a rehabilitation hospital, and the OTA trusts that a professional therapeutic relationship has been developed. The client then begins making indirect sexual comments to the OTA which they decide not to take seriously at the time. However, during the following week, the comments are becoming less discreet and more frequent. How should the OTA respond?

6. An OTA has been instructing a young adult client in a hand exercise program at the client's home following a sports injury. The client's father is well known in the community for owning and operating a popular winery. During a treatment session, the OTA happens to mention that they believe the supervising occupational therapist enjoys wine from the client's family winery, although the OTA actually prefers beer to wine. At the end of the following session, the client gives the OTA a bottle of award-winning wine, stating "you need to give this to the occupational therapist – my dad went to a lot of trouble to find our best wine for them." How does the OTA respond?

7. An OTA working in a hospital clinic has assisted the occupational therapist in fabricating a complicated hand splint for a client. When the client returns to the clinic ten days later following a physician appointment, they approach the OTA stating, "the surgeon wants my splint adjusted to increase the movement in my hand and asked that it could be completed as soon as possible." The occupational therapist who fabricated the splint is working in another clinic that week. How does the OTA respond?

8. A client was recently discharged from an occupational therapy treatment program in a private clinic. The OTA in the clinic provided treatment to assist with pain management as assigned by the occupational therapist and had developed a positive therapeutic relationship with the

client. A week following discharge, the client asks the OTA to "friend" them on Facebook. What does the OTA do?

9. The OTA has been visiting a client at home to improve independence with self-care activities and has developed a strong therapeutic relationship with both the client and her wife. During a recent visit, the client's wife shares with the OTA that she is concerned that her wife, the client, is not willing to take her medications, but she is afraid to tell the home care nurse in case her wife will be admitted to a nursing home. How does the OTA respond?

Ethical Decision-Making

How does an occupational therapist and/or an OTA approach ethical dilemmas within their practice as described in the previous examples?

Corbett describes a decision-making process that results in a "morally defensible decision as the most important outcome" (Corbett, 1993, p. 116). This process involves critical thinking and incorporates problem-solving into the decision making.

The steps within this process are as follows:

Identify the Problem	Clarify the issue and the underlying values influencing the problem.
Gather Data	Is there additional information that will assist in making the decision? Who is responsible for the action?
Identify Options	Map the various courses of action and the positive and negative consequence(s) of each action. Also consider the long-term implications for the actions and consequences identified.
Thinking through the Problem	Weigh each option against relevant obligations including applicable regulatory standards and code of ethics. What is the impact on everyone involved? Where is help or advice available?
Make a Decision	Determine the best course of action.
Act and Assess	Reviewing ethical decisions and their outcomes builds a personal data base.

(Corbett, 1993, pp. 116–117)

We will now return to the above examples and use this decision-making process to generate potential approaches from the author's perspective.

1. **An occupational therapist in a rural community has assessed a client following a motor vehicle accident. The occupational therapist has assigned an exercise program to the OTA who has recently moved back to this community. While reviewing the assignment, the OTA realizes that this client was a classmate ten years ago, and they have mutual friends. What does the OTA do?**

   • **Identify the problem**: The OTA has personal connections with a client to whom they have been assigned to provide occupational therapy treatment. This could affect the therapeutic relationship.

   • **Gather data**: Is there another OTA to whom this treatment could be assigned? The OTA will need to discuss this situation with the supervising occupational therapist.

   • **Identify options**:
      ▪ **A**. Assign to another OTA who does not have a personal relationship with the client.
      ▪ **B**. The occupational therapist delivers the treatment themselves.
      ▪ **C**. The OTA explains that although they know each other from high school, this is a therapeutic relationship between the OTA and the client.

   • **Thinking through the problem**:
      ▪ **A**. On review, there is no other OTA available so that is not an option.
      ▪ **B**. The therapist has a busy schedule, and although they are competent with the treatment, they would not be able to see the client as frequently as the OTA, therefore potentially affecting the client's outcome.
      ▪ **C**. The OTA is agreeable to treat the client but does not want to place the client in an uncomfortable situation.

- **Make a decision**: The decision is made by the therapist and the OTA to proceed with the initial assignment based on the client's agreement with the OTA providing the treatment.
- **Act and assess**: If the client does not agree with a former classmate being involved in providing therapy, the occupational therapist will provide the treatment as their schedule allows. If the client does agree and provides consent, the OTA will proceed with treatments and the outcomes will be evaluated, including the effectiveness of the OTA/client therapeutic relationship. The outcomes will also assist with future decision making in similar situations.

2. **A team colleague in a return-to-work clinical setting makes a racist comment in the staff room about an Indigenous client whom the OTA is also treating. The client experienced a shoulder dislocation following a work injury as a heavy-duty mechanic and is anxious to return to their job as soon as possible. What does the OTA do?**

   - **Identify the problem**: A healthcare professional has made a racist comment about a client. The OTA is the only person who heard the comment and knows that this is inappropriate even with the client not being present.
   - **Gather data**: The OTA recently completed a professional development course on improving how to communicate with Indigenous populations in healthcare environments and knows that anti-racism needs to be improved within their clinical setting. However, in this situation the team member is new to the staff and is also the OTA's supervisor with other clients. The therapist and OTA have not developed a strong therapeutic relationship as yet.
   - **Identify options**:
     - **A.** The OTA can tell the colleague that it is inappropriate to make racist comments about clients and also share information that they learned on their course.

- ■ **B**. The OTA can talk to their manager about the incident and how best to approach it.
- ■ **C**. The OTA can choose to not take any action.
- • **Thinking through the problem**:
    - ■ **A**. This is challenging for the OTA as the colleague may take offense and no longer assign client treatments to the OTA.
    - ■ **B**. Although this option could also upset the colleague by involving the manager, the OTA would benefit from the manager's recommendations as to how to deal with this situation.
    - ■ **C**. The OTA knows that taking no action is not the best decision to make, as anti-racism needs to be improved in the workplace.
- • **Make a decision**: The OTA decides to meet with the manager and following their discussion, the manager informs the OTA that they will bring up the topic of anti-racism at the next staff meeting. This will include information and processes about how to improve communication with and about Indigenous clients within their work setting.
- • **Act and assess**: The manager follows through on discussing the importance of improving anti-racism at the staff meeting and that outcomes will be reviewed regularly. Following the meeting, the OTA feels more comfortable bringing this topic up as needed in the future.

3. **An OTA is contracted at a complex care facility in a full-time position. The supervising occupational therapist is at the facility two days/week. The nurse approaches the OTA stating that the status of the resident in room 101 has declined over the past two days. The nurse then requests that the OTA contact the resident's daughter who is very involved in their mother's care. The daughter can then guide the OTA in any changes that need to be made to the occupational therapy treatment plan. How does the OTA respond?**
    - • **Identify the problem**: The nurse at the complex care facility is asking the OTA to act outside of their

responsibilities in discussing a resident's status with a family member.

- **Gather data**: The OTA can review the resident's health record documentation to better understand their status, as well as confirm with the nurse what specific functions have declined with the resident in the past two days.

- **Identify options**:
  - Visit the resident to continue with the assigned treatment program and report any observed changes to the supervising occupational therapist.
  - Place the treatment plan on hold and inform the supervising occupational therapist of the nurse's request.
  - The OTA could contact the resident's daughter but is uncomfortable with this decision.

- **Thinking through the problem**:
  - Continuing with the occupational therapy treatment program would likely not be the best option based on the nurse's concern.
  - Withholding the treatment would prevent the resident from receiving therapy, but the risks in continuing therapy could possibly be too high due to the resident's apparent declining status.
  - The OTA decides that contacting the resident's daughter as requested by the nurse is not within the OTA role.

- **Make a decision**: The best decision would be for the OTA to contact the supervising occupational therapist, or the alternate contact provided in the supervision plan in case of urgent situations if the therapist is not available. The OTA will discuss the issue, and then follow through on the recommendations. The assigned treatment would be discontinued until a new plan is in place. The OTA would also reinforce to the nurse that they cannot contact the resident's daughter to discuss changes in the therapy plan as that is the occupational therapist's role.

- **Act and assess**: After the decisions have been made and the treatment plan has been **changed** as needed by the occupational therapist, there would need to be further discussion with the care team at the facility as to the OTA's role and responsibilities including their limitations.

4. **The OTA has been treating a client following a back injury, and the occupational therapist is planning a reassessment to determine potential discharge by the end of the week. The client works as an accountant and has kindly offered to complete the OTA's tax return at a reduced cost. The deadline for filing the return is fast approaching and the OTA has not yet finished this task. How should the OTA respond?**
   - **Identify the problem**: The OTA has an opportunity to have their income tax return completed within the needed time frame at a more inexpensive cost, but this would result in the creation of a different relationship with the client.
   - **Gather data**: The client wants to show appreciation for the therapy provided by the OTA that has improved their occupational participation by completing the OTA's tax return at a decreased cost. The OTA is aware that this is likely not appropriate, but the tax deadline is quickly approaching.
   - **Identify options**:
     - The OTA agrees to proceed with the client's offer to complete their income tax return.
     - The OTA does not accept the offer as it would be ethically inappropriate.
   - **Thinking through the problem**:
     - This would create a power change in the relationship as the client would learn personal information about the OTA.
     - Although the OTA would need to find another way to complete their tax return, they would continue to have a therapeutic relationship with the client.

- **Make a decision**: The best decision is for the OTA not to accept the offer made by the client to complete their tax return.
- **Act and assess**: The OTA will inform the client in a professional manner that they cannot have the client complete their tax return. Based on this experience, the OTA will learn to be more aware of similar situations in the future and how to handle them.

5. **An OTA has been treating a client daily in a rehabilitation hospital, and the OTA trusts that a professional therapeutic relationship has been developed. The client then begins making indirect sexual comments to the OTA which they decide not to take seriously at the time. However, during the following week, the comments are becoming less discreet and more frequent. How should the OTA respond?**
   - **Identify the problem**: The client is crossing the professional relationship line by making sexual comments to the OTA who has been assigned to treat this client. These comments are increasing as the treatment proceeds.
   - **Gather data**: Although the OTA initially tries to ignore the sexual comments, they recognize this is inappropriate behavior by the client particularly when it is increasing and happening more frequently.
   - **Identify options**:
     - Inform the client that this is unacceptable behaviour which needs to stop so that the OTA can resume providing therapy in a professional manner.
     - Discuss the situation with the supervising occupational therapist to determine the best action to take.
   - **Thinking through the problem**:
     - The OTA's first option, if they are comfortable doing so, is to enter into a professional discussion with the client, stating that the sexual comments are inappropriate and they need to stop.

- ■ If the OTA is not comfortable with initiating this discussion, they will discuss their concerns with the occupational therapist and follow through with an agreed-upon approach. This may be that the occupational therapist will discuss the behaviors with the client and that they need to stop allowing the therapy to continue. It may also be best to assign this therapy treatment to another OTA if available.

- **Make a decision**: It would be best if the OTA is comfortable discussing this with the client, and then based on the client's response, potentially discuss it further with the supervising therapist.

- **Act and assess**: The agreed-upon plan will be put in place whether it is the OTA discussing this with the client, or the occupational therapist taking the lead. In the future, the OTA will have learned that as soon as this type of behavior begins with a client, it needs to be stopped right away to ensure that a professional relationship is maintained.

6. **An OTA has been instructing a young adult client in a hand exercise program at the client's home following a sports injury. The client's father is well known in the community for owning and operating a popular winery. During a treatment session, the OTA happens to mention that they believe the supervising occupational therapist enjoys wine from the client's family winery, although the OTA actually prefers beer to wine. At the end of the following session, the client gives the OTA a bottle of award-winning wine, stating "you need to give this to the occupational therapist – my dad went to a lot of trouble to find our best wine for them." How does the OTA respond?**

   - **Identify the problem**: The client has given the OTA a bottle of wine as a gift for the occupational therapist based on information provided by the OTA about the therapist enjoying the family's winery.

- **Gather data**: The OTA knows that the therapist would enjoy the wine but also is aware that **accepting** gifts from clients is unethical as it creates a more unprofessional relationship.
- **Identify options**:
  - The OTA can pass on the wine to the supervising occupational therapist and explain the situation.
  - The OTA can tell the client that they are not to accept gifts from clients and apologizes for giving the wrong message.
- **Thinking through the problem**: The best option is for the OTA not to accept the wine, although understands the client will be upset with this action.
- **Make a decision**: The best decision for the OTA to make is to not accept the wine for the therapist and explain to the client they are not to accept gifts.
- **Act and assess**: The OTA will follow up with this correct decision and be more aware in future client interactions to not engage in discussions related to potential gifts.

7. **An OTA working in a hospital clinic has assisted the occupational therapist in fabricating a complicated hand splint for a client. When the client returns to the clinic ten days later following a physician appointment, they approach the OTA stating, "the surgeon wants my splint adjusted to increase the movement in my hand and asked that it be completed as soon as possible." The occupational therapist who fabricated the splint is working in another clinic that week. How does the OTA respond?**
   - **Identify the problem**: The occupational therapist who fabricated the splint is not available at the clinic to make the adjustments requested by the surgeon as stated by the client, and this activity is outside of the OTA's responsibilities.
   - **Gather data**: The OTA understands that their role is not to adjust splint structure to this extent as it needs to be completed by the occupational therapist.

The occupational therapist will not return to work at the clinic for a week. There is another occupational therapist available, but the OTA is unsure of their knowledge with this type of splint.

- **Identify options:**
  - The OTA can try to contact the occupational therapist to explain the situation.
  - The OTA could discuss the situation with the other occupational therapist on site.
  - The OTA can ask the client to reach out to the occupational therapist and provide the client with the best contact information for the therapist.
- **Thinking through the problem**: Based on the OTA's understanding of their role within this situation, the most professional response would be to try to contact the occupational therapist themselves and explain the situation. However, the OTA is aware that the occupational therapist undertakes frequent client home visits while working at the other clinic and does not want to interrupt the therapist while working with a client in their home.
- **Make a decision**: The OTA decides to try to contact the occupational therapist and either discuss the situation in person or leave a voice mail and try to schedule another time to connect. As the OTA and the occupational therapist have developed a trusting professional relationship during their collaboration at the clinic, the OTA is confident that the occupational therapist will respect this decision.
- **Act and assess**: The OTA was able to connect with the occupational therapist. The occupational therapist asked the OTA to inform the client that the therapist would contact them later that day to discuss the situation and formulate a plan. The occupational therapist also planned to contact the surgeon to receive more information about their recommendation. Once the occupational therapist has completed the required splint adjustments to meet the client's goals, the OTA

and the therapist will review and evaluate this situation for similar events in the future.

8. **A client was recently discharged from an occupational therapy treatment program in a private clinic. The OTA in the clinic provided treatment to assist with pain management as assigned by the occupational therapist and had developed a positive therapeutic relationship with the client. A week following discharge, the client asks the OTA to "friend" them on Facebook. What does the OTA do?**

- **Identify the problem**: The OTA is asked by a recently discharged client to become a "friend" on Facebook which would change their therapeutic relationship to a more personal relationship.

- **Gather data**: The OTA understands that they are to maintain professional and therapeutic relationships with clients during treatment. However, now that the treatment is completed and the client is no longer attending the clinic, the OTA is unsure how to approach this situation as they do access Facebook on a regular basis.

- **Identify options**:
  - The OTA can discuss this situation with the supervising occupational therapist, although they know that the therapist does not use social media, and therefore may not provide an objective response.
  - The OTA could reach out to another colleague as to the best way to approach this type of situation.
  - The OTA can respond to the client that it is not appropriate, because the professional relationship just ended.
  - The OTA could simply not respond to the "friend" request.

- **Thinking through the problem**: Based on their understanding of professional relationships and ethical dilemmas learned from courses within their therapist assistant education program and during team information sessions within their workplace, the OTA feels uncomfortable making this decision without discussing with a colleague.

- **Make a decision**: The OTA reaches out to an occupational therapist who is on Facebook and asks for their opinion on how the OTA should respond to this situation. The therapist suggests that it is too early following discharge to connect with the client on social media.
- **Act and assess**: The OTA agrees with the therapist's suggestion and decides to not follow through on the request. If the client reached out again a year from now, the OTA may reconsider whether it would be appropriate after a longer period of time has passed.

9. **The OTA has been visiting a client at home to improve independence with self-care activities and has developed a strong therapeutic relationship with both the client and her wife. During a recent visit, the client's wife shares with the OTA that she is concerned that her wife, the client, is not willing to take her medications, but she is afraid to tell the home care nurse in case her wife will be admitted to a nursing home. How does the OTA respond?**

- **Identify the problem**: The client's wife is sharing a client health concern with the OTA that is unrelated to the assigned occupational therapy treatment plan.
- **Gather data**: The OTA could ask the client's wife how long this has been happening but, most importantly, the OTA would need to inform her that this information will have to be shared with the supervising occupational therapist, who will then discuss this further with her.
- **Identify options**: The OTA's only option in this situation is to ensure the client's wife understands that the OTA needs to inform the occupational therapist of this discussion, as it is beyond the OTA's responsibilities to make any decisions on this concern.
- **Thinking through the problem**: Although the client's wife may be uncomfortable with the OTA having to tell the therapist, it is a requirement of the OTA to follow through with informing the supervisor.

- **Make a decision**: The OTA will report this to the supervising occupational therapist as soon as possible.
- **Act and assess**: The OTA will inform the therapist who will be responsible for planning the best approach. This would likely involve discussing this situation further with the client's wife and encouraging her to talk to the home care nurse. The outcomes will then be evaluated. Based on this situation, the OTA will reinforce to future clients and their family members that health issues discussed with the OTA will need to be shared with the supervising therapist. If questions related to the assigned occupational therapy treatment are asked of the OTA, they can be answered or clarified by the assistant within the limitations of their treatment assignment.

Developing Trusting Relationships from the OTA Perspective

This section of the chapter was written by:

Debra Cooper, BAHSc., OTA & PTA
Toronto Rehabilitation Institute
Chair, CAOT OTA & PTA Practice Network

The role of an occupational therapist assistant (OTA) is often discussed or interpreted from the perspective of an occupational therapist. The following will discuss OTAs from the mindset of an assistant. OTAs are often excluded in role-related conversations about the clinical boundaries, abilities, or desires for growth within areas of practice pertaining to the OTA competencies. Ultimately, this leads to missed opportunities in building trusting and collaborative partnerships with therapists. Fortunately, with the release of the *Competencies for Occupational Therapists in Canada* (ACOTRO, ACOTUP, & CAOT, 2021) incorporating working with OTAs into the document, more assistants are being included in assignment discussions and clinical developments. Occupational therapists who collaborate closely with assistants develop an open and nurturing intraprofessional relationship which allows for the optimization of client performance.

Generally, OTAs are passionate clinicians and are well-versed in enhancing the provision of occupational therapy services to clients in various client populations. OTAs are highly skilled in exercising clinical judgment and treatment rationales and evaluating the therapeutic interventions that have been assigned. Assistants are valuable assets when it comes to the planning and execution of a client's goals. This is because they possess the clinical insights into providing secondary perspectives on not only how to meet the clinical objectives, but also how to individualize the care plan to the holistic needs of the client. Occupational therapists and OTAs share a compatible commitment to succeed when providing the best possible clinical interventions.

OTAs are able to support various practice areas in their assistance of therapists who work in clinical settings such as home care, private practice, and in acute and rehabilitation hospitals, either on inpatient care teams or within outpatient clinics. In recent years, more OTAs are being employed within the school systems, in mental health units, and providing virtual or remote care. Additionally, OTAs are able to play significant supporting roles within more specialized occupational therapy services, such as splinting or in wheelchair seating clinics. Assistants are able to work as self-employed individuals, meaning that they are able to seek out and accept contracts offered by occupational therapists, within the limitations of the OTA role. OTAs are not able to perform assessments, and therefore require the therapist to provide them with the assessment results and information about which impairments are to be treated. An example of this is transfer training education at a client's home. The occupational therapist is able to hire and contract out the task of teaching and practicing safe transfer training techniques. The OTA is accountable for supplying the supervising therapist with the correct documentation once the task is complete. As is the case with occupational therapists, the specific practice area in which an OTA primarily practices will influence clinical skills and knowledge base. However, assistants are adaptable and can adapt appropriately as client and therapist needs change. After all, OTAs are experts in providing hands-on therapeutic interventions as these skills are the core focus of many educational programs.

As the ever-changing service demands of healthcare increase the diversity of the occupational therapy scope, the occupational therapist and OTA collaborative partnership will be particularly important to clinical success. Historically, the role of the occupational therapist assistant has been misunderstood and is often subject to therapist-based biases as a result. OTAs knowingly work within set clinical competencies and are able to gauge the boundaries of their abilities while simultaneously knowing how to expand clinical opportunities under the supervision of an occupational therapist.

Benefits of a Clinical Partnership from an OTA Lens

Undoubtedly, the positive impact on client care is the most beneficial aspect of the partnership between occupational therapists and occupational therapist assistants. Assistants should be viewed as an extension of the therapist, as collaborative care partners and as an equal contributor to treatment planning. OTA training and experience equips them with the ability to provide valuable clinical insights and treatment rationales that are catered to an individual client's needs. Incorporating assistants into the care plan allows for an increase not only in available time for face-to-face interventions, but also in the variety of treatment opportunities that can be provided. Consider task assignment discussions as an example: if working towards the same goal, electing which activities both the therapist and the assistant will focus on; if working towards multiple goals, deciding who is going to focus on which one. Alternatively, if the OTA's assignment is preparing the client for the therapist's session by implementing modalities, like paraffin wax on hands, or stretching, this allows for improved efficiency and allotted intervention time for more complex activities. Working with an OTA also provides the opportunity to participate in a joint or co-treatment session with clients, allowing for more challenging and creative treatment implementation and planning.

An additional benefit to working with OTAs is the different perspective that is offered to the therapeutic dynamic. Experientially, as a result of many different factors, OTAs tend to be of increased diversity in comparison with occupational therapists. Divergent influences that contribute to OTA diversity may include ethnicity, cultural or, religious belief, educational backgrounds, or socioeconomic circumstances. These conditions should be considered when approaching an assistant to begin and then also to maintain a strong working partnership. It is recommended to remain mindful of the existence of barriers that OTAs often confront when selecting a career path or upgrading to becoming a therapist. Obstacles in accessing education are not limited to the assistant group but include financial means and familial responsibilities as primary hurdles. In some circumstances, an OTA may be internationally trained as an occupational therapist, but does not have the credentials to practice in Canada. From a different perspective, these characteristics are generally advantageous while building client rapport, as it subconsciously deems the OTAs as more relatable, resulting in stronger therapeutic connections. Occupational therapists should recognize this exchange as a benefit and incorporate it into practice as the Canadian healthcare system continues to evolve and services are becoming more limited due to the lack of available resources.

Barriers to Building Clinical Partnerships from an OTA Lens

Occupational therapy, like all professions, is constantly evolving as it works in compliance with the healthcare needs of the Canadian population. The scope of practice is continually broadening and the demands to optimize client care are expected given strained resources. Additionally, there are challenges within the intraprofessional partnership between occupational therapists and OTAs. The word "assistant" attracts subconscious bias which can inadvertently become the third party within the working dynamics of therapists and assistants. Unfortunately, there are discrepancies between the professions in acknowledging that controversy exists. From the perspective of an OTA, misunderstandings about the assistant role, clinical competencies, and training are contributing factors. While working with OTAs, therapists need to be cognizant about how to approach the clinical partnership, with diversification at the forefront. It is important to consider elements such as cultural differences, including language barriers, ethnicity, and socioeconomic circumstances, simply as individualized qualities and to not underestimate an assistant's abilities because of them. Affordability, external responsibilities, and available time are often barriers as to why an OTA has not pursued a master's degree in occupational therapy; it is not a question of intelligence.

The same barriers that can prevent occupational therapists and OTAs from forming concrete collaborative partnerships also simultaneously contribute to power differentials within the relationship. As assistants work under the supervision of occupational therapists, it is the therapist's responsibility to maintain a sense of equity within the working partnership. By having this balance, the opportunity for creating psychological safer spaces for both therapist and assistant is possible. Not having the option for mutually safer spaces can lead to missed collaborative opportunities to enhance client care, assigning inappropriate tasks to OTAs, and risking client harm if the assistants do not feel comfortable about asking clarifying questions. If an assistant does not feel they are viewed as an equal partner within the working relationship, they are much less likely to speak up regarding practice concerns in fear of the repercussions.

Understanding the Benefits of Dual-Trained Assistants

In Canada, OTAs are commonly dual trained as physiotherapist assistants (PTAs). However, in some provinces assistants may also have training in speech and language pathology or therapeutic recreation. Assistants are comfortable switching their practice focus depending on the discipline being assigned. OTAs are able to demonstrate understanding and critical thinking concerning how to perform tasks or problem-solve using both occupational therapy and physiotherapy practice lenses at the same time. A major advantage to the dual training is the ability to comprehend dual goals, allowing for the assistant to complement each therapeutic objective and combining them to a joint profession treatment session. Occupational therapists have the opportunity to further collaborate with physiotherapists by creating dual referrals for efficiency in achieving similar or complementary goals. An example of dual referrals is ambulation and wayfinding or bed-mobility and dressing activities for daily living. OTAs are also able to act as a direct link to the patient's physiotherapy goals and current interventions, enabling a more holistic and client-centered clinical approach. It is important to note that some assistants appear to be stronger in physiotherapy-type physical interventions. These assistants may be well-suited for more remedial upper extremity programs or physical treatment plans; however, this does not mean that these assistants lack the necessary skills to perform cognitive retraining or other occupational therapy tasks. It is important to note that dual-trained assistants are expected to know the role differentiation between the disciplines that initiate each referral. Assistants are to report discipline-related practice concerns to the correct avenue; more specifically, OTA-related issues must be voiced to the supervising occupational therapist and PTA matters to the supervising physiotherapist.

Differences in How to Work with a New OTA vs. an Experienced OTA

Working with and incorporating OTAs into clinical practice can be intimidating for occupational therapists when entering the workforce or a new practice area, particularly when encountering a very skilled or experienced assistant within any practice area. As a new occupational therapist graduate, it is important to consider the advantageous collaborative and learning opportunities that can present themselves by working together. Lived experiences are a significant aspect to the development of critical thinking and reflective practice, which cannot be taught in a vocational setting. Experienced OTAs are a valuable resource for treatment planning, problem-solving, and creatively integrating the holistic individual needs of each client into therapeutic interventions. A newly practicing occupational therapist having transparency with developing specific clinical skills and demonstrating vulnerability to learning from an assistant will have a positive impact on the future therapeutic partnership. Assistants will view this gesture as respectful and will appreciate the recognition. Additionally, asking for OTA support is an excellent opportunity for guidance and mentorship; it does not lessen a therapist's contributions to clinical care but strengthens collaborative care planning.

An advantage to working with a newly graduated OTA, or one moving to a new practice area, is mutual learning. As is the case with occupational therapists, it is not possible for assistants to gain exposure to every clinical setting while in training; however, the fundamental knowledge base is available to expand upon. The opportunity for mutual learning and clinical development will guide cohesion within the therapist and assistant partnership. It is a fantastic opportunity to create a working dynamic that is mutually beneficial and will help with guiding coherent clinical care approaches. As in any new working relationship, trial and error is a part of the process and to be expected. It is advisable to have continual discussions to determine that each member's needs are being addressed and met. A similar approach is beneficial when moving into new practice areas or workplace settings. Despite experience levels, OTAs possess transferable skills that can be adapted to better support a therapist's caseload and optimize client care.

Strategies to Building Stronger Trusting Partnerships

Building a strong and trusting relationship is crucial to having a successful occupational therapist and OTA collaborative partnership. Spending time together is necessary to create mutual understanding and a supportive working alliance. The following strategies are guidelines to help develop connections between the professions.

◆ **Discover each other's strengths**
  A great starting point to working with a new assistant is to learn about each other's clinical strengths and interests. Through discussion and observation, aim to establish the skills that an OTA colleague is comfortable performing and discover the specific therapeutic interventions they are passionate about. Learning about the experiences an assistant has had within different client populations will also help with treatment planning and task assignments. Education and additional professional development courses are valid topics of conversations to gain clarity on the individual assistant's role and training. It is important to reflect on and remove any unconscious

biases during this process, as assistant diversity is a clinical benefit and a strength in healthcare teams.

◆ **View an OTA colleague as a care partner**

By treating an OTA as a clinical care partner rather than just being an "assistant" will have a positive impact on clinical interventions. Communicating client goals, progress, and treatment planning openly with an assistant will better support the client's needs, allowing for additional therapeutic contributions and execution of the occupational therapist's vision. Inclusion in family meeting and care rounds is within the OTA professional abilities and provides the opportunity to demonstrate how occupational therapy is supporting a client's recovery. On an intraprofessional and interprofessional platform it is important to emphasize that OTAs are an extension of occupational therapy services, both interprofessionally to team members and intraprofessionally to clients and their families, during clinical interactions. Maintaining a trustworthy dynamic and partnership will enable reciprocal development and professional growth.

◆ **Collaborate together**

OTAs are resourceful and valuable allies when it comes to client care and the promotion of occupational therapy services and delivery. By having a different perspective and approach to client care, assistants are able to provide insights and opinions and contribute effectively to treatment planning. By asking an OTA about the experiences with a specific client or to share any observations will not only enrich the client's experience, but also allow for the client's recovery potential to be increased through additional therapeutic intervention. Planning joint or co-treatment sessions with an OTA presents another fantastic opportunity to problem-solve while optimizing each other's clinical skill sets. As previously mentioned, OTAs are often physiotherapy assistants as well. The dual lens enables interprofessional understanding to be incorporated into the client's treatment session and how to achieve the targeted occupational therapy goals simultaneously.

◆ **Initiating joint treatment sessions**

Understandably, learning how to work with OTAs effectively can be a stressful experience for occupational therapists. Developing joint or co-treatment sessions is an essential tool in showcasing mutual clinical skills and as a team-building initiative. Scheduling time together is not only an appropriate strategy for an OTA to transparently demonstrate their clinical skills, but also an opportunity to ask clarifying questions for both parties involved. Additionally, it will allow the occupational therapist to demonstrate clinic skill expectations to the assistant prior to task assignment. It is advisable to remain mindful of how feedback is provided and to learn which communication style would be most complementary to building partnerships, while avoiding inadvertently displaying a professional power differential. By including assistants in the treatment planning process, an occupational therapist will have the opportunity to discover the depth of an assistant's abilities to critically think and provide treatment rationales. Further allowing the therapist and assistant to create treatment plans will complement clinical strengths, encourage areas of desired growth and mutual professional development interest, while optimizing clinical care.

Explore Role-Emerging Assignments

The term role-emerging was traditionally used when discussing innovative student fieldwork placements; however, it has since been broadened to incorporate new or nontraditional OTA roles. Naturally, as the occupational therapy profession expands into more unconventional areas of practice, assistant roles need to be developed to support the need.

Creating a position designed for an OTA allows for a therapist to truly gain the required clinical support for the specific demands of that particular area of practice. Having an open discussion with an OTA during the creation of the role will enable dual perspectives to best encompass each other's knowledge, clinical skill sets, and innovative conceptualization. OTAs know the capacities and limitations set out in the *Competencies for Occupational Therapist Assistants* document. (CAOT, 2024). Better outcomes will be met during position creation when assistants and therapists work together as partners, in a trusting environment, allowing for mutual trial and error during the creative and evaluation process.

This concept is included in the online module, *Working Together for Optimal Outcomes: Occupational Therapists and OT-Assistants in Canada* (Avvampato, Finlayson, Fong-Lee, Hall, 2023).

OTA Interactions in Fieldwork Placements

Occupational therapists' fieldwork placements provide an excellent opportunity to practice clinical interactions with OTAs. The specific workplace setting will impact the types of therapeutic interventions and required supports that OTAs are involved with. Either way, it is an opportunity to train in communication and supervision strategies, performing in joint treatment sessions, and in how and what tasks to assign. Assistants are often very willing to work with student occupational therapists and appreciate being approached to provide guidance and clinical expertise from an OTA's perspective. Having these exposures in a safe learning environment will make for a more seamless transition to a working partnership after graduation. Additionally, clarity can be gained on the occupational therapist assistant competencies and how they align to those of an occupational therapist, which will help facilitate a stronger collaborative partnership in the future.

Negative Impacts of Not Building OTA Partnerships

Not working towards a collaborative partnership with OTAs has a negative impact which greatly influences the quality of client care being provided. Misunderstandings of the OTA role within the occupational therapy profession result in unnecessary mutual frustrations and tension between assistants and therapists. Without having the correct tools to accurately build a strong collaborative partnership, the quality of care provided will reflect the consequences of the missed opportunities. Therapists are further at risk of caregiver burnout and feelings of being overwhelmed as the healthcare demands change with the evolution of client needs.

If therapists and assistants do not create a mutually psychologically safe working dynamic, true collaborative practice cannot occur. Assistants are an extension of the occupational therapist and, like any good relationship, mutual respect and understanding are needed to maintain a successful partnership. Not only will this make work more effective and productive, and increase the quality of care provided, it will also be more enjoyable for all those involved. Embrace mutual advocacy and the collaborative possibilities can be endless.

Reflections on Intraprofessional and Interprofessional Relationships

This chapter has so far discussed many positive and also concerning factors related to intraprofessional and interprofessional therapeutic relationships. It is critical that trusting relationships be developed within a healthcare team, whether between an occupational therapist and an OTA, an occupational therapist and a physiotherapist, or a manager and the team for which they are responsible.

Depending on their current or future roles, readers are encouraged to consider the following situations and reflect on how to develop or improve professional relationships within their therapy setting.

- ◆ **Occupational therapists**: Reflect on a process you could initiate to build intraprofessional relationships with OTA(s) whom you have not previously collaborated with during client treatments. In addition, consider ways that you could improve existing relationships with OTAs to increase an understanding of their competence.
- ◆ **OTAs**: Reflect on how you would encourage new occupational therapists, or occupational therapists you have not previously collaborated with in your work environment, to initiate building trusting intraprofessional relationships – or how this could be initiated if you relocated to a new work environment. In addition, consider possible opportunities for increasing the therapists' understanding of your skills and knowledge.
- ◆ **Managers/leaders within therapy settings**: Reflect on how you would support and enable your team members to develop both intraprofessional and interprofessional relationships through professional development education opportunities, mentoring, or other possibilities.

Frequently Asked Questions

1. **When an OTA's previous role in healthcare was as a care aide, what does the OTA need to understand about working in their new role within the same work environment?** The OTA needs to understand that this is a different role and that they now work under the direction and supervision of the occupational therapist, not the nurse as in their

previous role. If a nurse approaches the OTA to ask them to perform a specific care task for a client to whom they are providing occupational therapy, the OTA needs to be sufficiently self-confident to explain to the nurse that even though they used to work under the nurse's direction, they are now in a new career and cannot perform this task. The OTA may be able to incorporate previous skills learned when working as a care aide but the situation would need to be discussed first with the supervising occupational therapist, and the therapist would have to agree. In most situations, an OTA would not be able to apply care aide skills within their therapist assistant role as it is outside of the occupational therapy scope. An example of this is as follows:

- The OTA is teaching a client ambulation using a new four-wheeled walker followed by practicing transfers on and off the toilet. During one of the treatment sessions, the client is not able to control their bowels prior to reaching the toilet and experiences faecal incontinence. This personal care incident requires the client to receive peri care, which the OTA is competent to perform. However, as it outside of the OTA role and there is a risk of affecting skin integrity, the OTA would need to contact the care aide or nurse who is responsible for the client and explain the situation that occurred. The care aide or nurse would then provide the peri care, and the OTA would include this occurrence within their health record documentation.

2. **If an OTA previously worked as an education assistant within the school system, what understandings do they need to have about their new OTA role?**

The OTA needs to understand that they perform treatments only assigned by the supervising occupational therapist. The tasks may be similar to activities they completed as an education assistant, but the specific requirements, frequency, and methods will be under the direction and supervision of the occupational therapist. This process must also be understood by the teacher of the student the OTA is treating, as well as by the student's parents.

3. **What are the benefit and outcomes of learning effective communication skills within the occupational therapist and OTA relationship?**

Effective communication is critical in all relationships including collaborative relationships within a workplace, particularly when one person in the relationship is accountable for the work performed by another team member. In this relationship, the occupational therapist is responsible for safe and effective therapy to be consistently provided to their clients including when they have assigned treatments to OTAs. It is the responsibility of the OTA to regularly communicate with the supervising occupational therapist as to the client's status, progress, challenges, and outcomes in addition to communicating appropriately with the clients as to their OTA role. Therefore, effective communication between the occupational therapist and the OTA is an essential component of the relationship to ensure optimal benefits for the clients.

Domain B, Communication *and Collaboration*, within both the *Competencies for Occupational Therapists in Canada 2021* and the *Competencies for OTAs 2024*, states:

The competent occupational therapist is expected to: *and*

The competent OTA is expected to:

◆ **B1 Communicate in a respectful and effective manner**
  • **B1.1** Organize thoughts, prepare content, and present professional views clearly.
  • **B1.2** Foster the successful exchange of information to develop mutual understanding.
  • **B1.3** Employ communication approaches and technologies suited to the context and client needs (specifically verbal, nonverbal, and written).

- **B1.4** Adjust to power imbalances that affect relationships and communication.

> (ACOTRO, ACOTUP, CAOT, 2021,
> p. 12; CAOT, 2024, p. 9)

The competent OTA is expected to:

- **B1.5** Recognize and communicate with clients and other professionals the limits of the OTA role.

> (CAOT, 2024, p. 9)

These *competencies* reinforce the importance of communication within the occupational therapist and OTA relationship in addition to therapeutic relationships with the clients and interprofessional relationships with other team members.

4. **How does building a trusting intraprofessional relationship between an occupational therapist and an OTA impact the clients?**

An occupational therapist and OTA trusting relationship will provide consistent flow throughout the client's treatments. Both the therapist and the assistant will be confident in communicating with each other if the client has questions and/or if any ethical dilemmas occur.

Certain issues that may arise during the treatment sessions may require therapist and OTA collaboration to effectively problem-solve the issue. This joint service provision "enables further development of mutual trust and problem solving to address the clients' needs" (McCready-Wirth, Hepting, Ng, Haney, Bratkoski, & MacAusland-Berg, 2015, p. 19). The OTA will also be comfortable initiating a discussion with the supervising therapist about a different approach or tool they could incorporate in this client's treatment, based on the OTA's previous experience with another client presenting with similar functional limitations.

Examples of these client situations could include the following:

1. A client has skin breakdown on her heels which is initially thought to be caused by pressure while the client is lying in bed. However, through joint problem-solving by the occupational therapist and the OTA, it was determined the skin breakdown was the result of the client self-propelling their wheelchair in bare feet with the heels rubbing on the hub of the axle and the footplates. The offending parts of the wheelchair were then padded, which resulted in eventual healing of the wound ((McCready-Wirth, Hepting, Ng, Haney, Bratkoski, & MacAusland-Berg, 2015, p. 20).

2. A client requires cognitive training to address specific limitations they are experiencing. The occupational therapist is unsure of the resources available within their workplace that would address this issue. In a collaborative discussion, the OTA informed the therapist they had previously worked with a client demonstrating similar cognitive limitations and had created a cognitive resource tool which resulted in a positive outcome for that client. Upon review of the resource, the therapist agreed this would be a beneficial treatment tool for their client and, following reassessment after a two-week treatment period, the client demonstrated improved cognitive function.

The optimal outcome of building this trusting relationship will provide a positive and respectful treatment experience for the client. This will increase the potential for the client to meet their goals and increase their quality of life. This collaboration is reflected in Domain B, *Communication and Collaboration*, in the *Competencies for Occupational Therapist Assistants*, within the following indicators:

The competent OTA is expected to:

♦ **B3 Collaborate with supervising occupational therapist(s) and clients**

- **B3.1** Partner with clients in decision making.
- **B3.2** Share information about the OTA role and knowledge.
- **B3.3** Identify practice situations that would benefit from collaborative care.
- **B3.4** Maintain mutually supportive working relationships.
- **B3.5** Participate actively and respectfully in collaborative decision making.
- **B3.6** Participate in team evaluation and improvement initiatives.
- **B3.7** Support evidence-informed team decision making.
- **B3.8** Address real or potential conflict in a fair, respectful, supportive, and timely manner.

(CAOT, 2024, p. 8)

This competency and indicators reinforce that intraprofessional collaboration in addition to collaboration with the clients is necessary for effective client outcomes within all work environments.

5. **How does an occupational therapist and OTA relationship develop in a virtual setting when an OTA is located in one location and the therapist is in another location, potentially a far distance away?**
This can be challenging, as was shared by Bellefontaine, Hurley, and Irngaut in their 2015 article. The OTA, or CTA as titled in the article, works in a northern community that is far from where the supervising occupational therapists are located. "The distance alone delays information sharing and limits opportunities for timely feedback, direct skill transfer and spontaneous collaboration" (Bellefontaine, Hurley, & Irngaut, 2015, p. 22). However, the occupational therapist and CTA relationship has developed during the therapist's in-person client visits and as the CTA is a member of the community, she has been able to "act as a language interpreter" and also "supports these therapists, who have relocated to this

region from southern parts of Canada, to develop a more nuanced understanding of local practices and knowledge in relation to health and health care" (Bellefontaine, Hurley, & Irngaut, 2015, p. 21).

It is best if the occupational therapist and OTA relationship can be developed in person, but when this is not possible, the partnership can be established through the use of technology. This can include phone conversations and the therapist can observe the OTA providing interventions via video connections followed by communication with the OTA when the treatment is completed. This virtual type of connection became more accepted during COVID-19 and although it does not replace in-person collaborations, it is definitely an option to consider.

References

Association of Canadian Occupational Therapy Regulatory Organizations, Association of Canadian Occupational Therapy University Programs, & Canadian Association of Occupational Therapists. (2021). *Competencies for occupational therapists in Canada.* OT-Competency-Document-EN-HiRes.pdf (acotro-acore.org)

Avvampato, T., Finlayson, M., Fong-Lee, D., & Hall, M. (2023). *Working together for optimal outcomes: Occupational therapists and OT-assistants in Canada* [online]. Licensed under CC BY-NC-ND 4.0. https://ot-ota-collaboration-resource-link.tiiny.co

Bellefontaine, K., Hurley, M., & Irngaut, S. (2015). Community therapy assistant: Supporting rehabilitation services in the remote arctic community of Igloolik, Nunavut. *Occupational Therapy Now, 17*(2), 21–22.

Canadian Association of Occupational Therapists. (2018). *Code of ethics.* https://caot.in1touch.org/document/4604/codeofethics.pdf

Canadian Association of Occupational Therapists. (2024). *Competencies for occupational therapist assistants.* https://caot.ca/document/8146/Competencies%20OTA%20EN%20Feb%208%202024.pdf

Corbett, K. (1993). Ethics and occupational therapy practice. *Canadian Journal of Occupational Therapy, 60*(3), 115–117.

Donnellan, L. & Gerlach, A. (2018). *Exploring acute care occupational therapists' & therapy assistants' collaborative practices. CAOT Conference Presentation 2018.* Vancouver, BC.

Etty, S., Snaith, B., Hinchcliffe, D., & Nightingale, J. (2024). The deployment and utilization of the Allied Health Professions Support Workforce: A scoping review. *Journal of Multidisciplinary Healthcare, 17,* 2251–2269.

Francis, D. & Strader, C. (2015). The role of occupational therapist assistant and physiotherapist assistant students on an interprofessional education unit. *Occupational Therapy Now, 17*(2), 29–30.

Gerber, S. (2022). *Emotional magnetism: How to communicate to ignite connection in your relationships.* Vancouver: NEXT IMPACT Press.

Gillespie, H. (2023). Occupational therapist and OTA collaboration: The how is now. *Occupational Therapy Now, 26*(6), 9–12.

Gillespie, H. & Engel, L. (2015). Occupational therapist assistants: Enabling well-being in community power mobility users. *Occupational Therapy Now, 17*(2), 8–10.

Hagler, P., Madill, H., & Kennedy, L. (1994). Facing choices about our beliefs regarding support personnel. *Canadian Journal of Occupational Therapy, 61*(4), 215–218.

McCready-Wirth, A., Hepting, C., Ng, W., Haney, C., Bratkoski, L., & MacAusland-Berg, D. (2015). On the road together: Community occupational therapists and occupational therapist assistants working to provide the best care. *Occupational Therapy Now, 17*(2), 19–20.

Penner, J., Snively, A., Packham, T., Henderson, J., Principi, E., & Malstrom, B. (2020). Viewpoints of the occupational therapist assistant – Physiotherapist assistant role on inter-professional teams: A mixed-methods study. *Physiotherapy Canada, 72*(4), 394–405. https://doi.org/10.3138/ptc-2019-0011

Stephenson, J. (2015). Working together: Today's dynamic duo! *Occupational Therapy Now, 17*(2), 28.

World Federation of Occupational Therapists. (2024). *Guiding principles for ethical occupational therapy.* https://wfot.org/resources/wfot-guiding-principles-for-ethical-occupational-therapy

3

Assignment and Supervision

Objectives

After completing this chapter, the reader will be able to:

- ◆ Describe the difference between assignment, delegation, and consultation.
- ◆ Understand applicable provincial regulation requirements for utilizing OTAs within occupational therapy service delivery.
- ◆ Recognize task examples that can potentially be assigned to OTAs.
- ◆ Understand effective decision-making processes to determine assignment of task to OTAs.
- ◆ Describe types of supervision and when each is required.
- ◆ Recognize components of a supervision and communication plan.

Key Terms

- ◆ Assignment
- ◆ Delegation
- ◆ Consultation
- ◆ Occupational participation
- ◆ Assignment decision-making process
- ◆ Supervision

DOI: 10.4324/9781003498391-3

- ◆ Communication
- ◆ Documentation
- ◆ Professional liability insurance

Frequently Asked Questions (FAQs) are included at the end of this chapter.

Provincial Regulation for Task Assignment

The Association of Canadian Occupational Therapy Regulatory Organizations (ACOTRO) published a position statement in 2019 titled *Utilizing Occupational Therapist Assistants in Occupational Therapy Service Delivery*. Although each province has regulatory documents related to Assignment and Supervision of OTAs, this position statement provides a general understanding of the occupational therapist/OTA collaboration and will be referenced throughout this chapter (ACOTRO, 2019). Occupational therapists are currently not regulated in Yukon, Northwest Territories, or Nunavut.

It is imperative that occupational therapists review the guideline/standard related to assignment and supervision of OTAs within their province and contact the respective College with any questions and/or to ask for clarification as needed. It is also important that OTAs review these documents to ensure their understanding of the assignment and supervision requirements that the occupational therapists must follow.

The Association of Canadian Occupational Therapy Regulatory Organizations, or ACOTRO, provides information and links to each Occupational Therapy Regulator within their website: https://acotro-acore.org/.

Assignment or Delegation?

The terms "assignment" and "delegation" have been used interchangeably over the years. Previously, it was not of significant concern but that has now changed in healthcare. Currently, within some provinces, the term "delegation" is specific to delegation of a regulated activity, restricted act, or controlled act to another provider (ACOTRO, 2019). Therefore, occupational therapy treatments or service components are "assigned" to OTAs, not "delegated." The use of "assignment" to OTAs must be consistent in all clinical settings across the country to ensure the understanding of involving OTAs within occupational therapy service delivery.

To Assign or Not to Assign?

This can be a challenging question, particularly for therapists who have had no or limited experience working with OTAs. As referred to in Chapter 1, Domain A, *Occupational Therapy Expertise*, in the 2021 *Competencies for Occupational Therapists in Canada* states the following:

The competent occupational therapist is expected to:

◆ **A7 Manage the assignment of services to assistants and others**
  - **A7.1** Identify practice situations where clients may benefit from services assigned to assistants or others.
  - **A7.2** Assign services only to assistants and others who are competent to deliver services.
  - **A7.3** Monitor the safety and effectiveness of assignments through supervision, mentoring, teaching, and coaching.
  - **A7.4** Follow the regulatory guidance for assigning and supervising services.
                         (ACOTRO, ACOTUP, CAOT 2021, p. 11)

It will be re-emphasized here that occupational therapists need to refer to their Regulatory College document that outlines pertinent assignment responsibilities and supervision requirements, and to contact their College when they require further clarification. The ACOTRO Position Statement (2019) describes the general role of the occupational therapist when utilizing assistants to deliver occupational therapy services as follows:

1. Initiation of occupational therapy services
2. Conducting occupational therapy assessments especially when clinical judgment is required

3. Interpretation of assessments
4. Intervention planning and goal setting
5. Communication requiring clinical judgment
6. Discharge decisions/planning
7. Determining if assignment of occupational therapy services components to assistants is appropriate and related to intervention plans and goals.

(ACOTRO, 2019, p. 1)

Tasks that are not to be assigned by the occupational therapist include:

♦ Treatments requiring ongoing analysis by an occupational therapist.
♦ Occupational therapy components that the occupational therapist is not competent to direct.
♦ Modifying interventions beyond what is established by the supervising occupational therapist.
♦ Referral to other professions or agencies.
♦ Communications of occupational therapy recommendations, opinions, findings.

OTA Role

As previously discussed, the role of the OTA is to carry out the intervention plans assigned to them by an occupational therapist and to represent themselves as an assistant working under the occupational therapist's direction/supervision. This will ensure clarity that OTAs do not work independently (ACOTRO, 2019).

The CAOT *Competencies for Occupational Therapist Assistants* within Domain A, *Occupational Therapist Assistant Expertise*, state that:

The competent OTA is expected to:

♦ **A2 Facilitate occupational participation in a range of practice contexts**
  • **A2.1** Keep the clients' occupations at the centre of practice

- **A2.2** Demonstrate understanding of the client's occupational therapy plan
- **A2.3** Implement assigned service components of the occupational therapy plan
- **A2.4** Observe, monitor, document, and report the client's performance
- **A2.5** Facilitate clients' use of their strengths and resources to sustain occupational participation
- **A2.6** Work effectively with individuals, families, and groups
- **A2.7** Complete assigned data gathering elements using a range of tools to support the occupational therapy evaluation process.

(CAOT, 2024, p. 7)

These indicators within this competency will be discussed and referenced in more detail throughout this chapter.

The *Competencies for Occupational Therapist Assistants* also state within Domain E, *Professional Responsibility*, that "OTAs are responsible for safe, ethical, and effective practice. They maintain high standards of occupational therapy practice and work in the best interests of clients and society" (CAOT, 2024, p.11).

This is described in further detail by stating:

The competent OTA is expected to:

- ◆ **E1 Work within the legislative and regulatory requirements for occupational therapists**
  - **E1.1** Respect the laws, codes of ethics, rules, and regulations that govern occupational therapy.
  - **E1.2** Work within personal competence and limits of assigned task.
  - **E1.3** Obtain and maintain informed consent in a way that is appropriate for the practice context.
  - **E1.4** Protect client privacy and confidentiality.
  - **E1.5** Respond to ethical dilemmas based on ethical frameworks and client values.
  - **E1.6** Take action with supervising occupational therapist(s) to manage their own real or potential *conflicts of interest*.

- **E1.7** Be accountable for all of their own decisions and actions made in the course of practice.
- **E1.8** Respond to and report observed unprofessional, unethical, or oppressive behaviour, as required.
- **E1.9** Respect professional boundaries by maintaining effective collaborative relationships with clients and team members.

◆ **E2 Demonstrate a commitment to minimizing risk**

- **E2.1** Follow organizational policies and procedures and take action if they are in conflict with professional standards, client values, practice evidence, or protocols.
- **E2.2** Respect clients' *occupational rights* and choices while minimizing risks.
- **E2.3** Take preventive measures to reduce risks to self-clients, and the public.

(CAOT, 2024, p. 11)

This competency needs to be clearly understood by OTAs to ensure that safe, ethical, and effective occupational therapy treatments are provided to clients by OTAs. Although OTAs are not regulated, they need to understand the regulatory requirements that their supervising occupational therapists must follow based on their provincial registration.

What Tasks Can Be Assigned to an OTA?

This is a common question and the answer in most situations is that any occupational therapy treatment can be assigned based on level of risk resulting from working through the decision to assign process that is discussed below. It must be mentioned here that if an occupational therapy treatment is listed as a restricted or protected activity within the pertinent occupational therapy regulator organization, it cannot be assigned to an OTA.

Occupational therapists are often looking for a "cookie-cutter" approach when determining what treatment can be assigned to an OTA for clients with a particular condition, diagnosis, or clinical situation. For example, the same occupational therapy treatment protocol will be assigned for any client who is recovering from a total hip replacement surgery with similar supervision plans incorporated into the plan. However, this is often not a safe or effective method to apply as every client has various treatment requisites based on their individual co-morbidities, environmental contexts, and cultural needs. In addition, each OTA demonstrates various skill competencies, and it cannot be assumed that each OTA can perform all assigned treatments. This leads to the importance of utilizing a decision-making process in determining whether to assign or the ways to assign client treatments to OTAs. This process will be discussed later in the chapter.

Certain potential tasks that may be assigned to OTAs as direct client care treatments are described below within certain categories, and these treatments can be applied in various clinical environments. Keep in mind that this is definitely not an exhaustive list, but the intention is to provide insight into potential options for readers to consider within their individual work settings.

Assisting the Occupational Therapist in an Assessment or Collaborating Within a Treatment Session

◆ Setting up the environment with required equipment and assistive devices prior to the assessment or treatment session being completed by the occupational therapist.

◆ Supporting the client's limb during splint fabrication by the occupational therapist.

◆ Assisting the therapist with transfer assessment or practice if the client's stability fluctuates.

◆ Pushing a wheelchair behind a client who is learning to ambulate using a new mobility device through instruction by the therapist.

◆ Co-facilitating a support group for clients with bipolar disorder.

◆ Assisting the occupational therapist during a client's wheelchair assessment by adjusting the wheelchair as the therapist determines the appropriate fit to meet the client's needs.

◆ Problem-solving with a therapist to determine the cause of a particular issue or the best treatment option in a specific situation.

Implementing Client Treatment Following an Assignment and Supervision Plan

◆ Teaching a hand exercise program to a client following a work injury.

◆ Completing splint fabrication by adding straps and adjusting the splint as needed.

◆ Guiding the client to safely and confidently reintegrate back into the community following a mental health crisis.

◆ Assisting the client to become independent with dressing activities using assistive devices as needed.

◆ Adjusting a pressure-relieving cushion such as ROHO to assist in healing a pressure sore.

◆ Training the client to safely operate a power mobility device within the community.

◆ Teaching, adapting, and/or grading a specific leisure activity in which the client is motivated to participate.

◆ Assisting a long-term care resident with feeding tasks by teaching them to use adaptive utensils.

◆ Teaching the client cognitive retraining activities following a traumatic brain injury.

◆ Assisting a child exhibiting issues with fine motor skills to develop handwriting abilities.

◆ Teaching a client with an acquired brain injury the steps involved in the task of showering.

◆ Assisting a client with dementia to perform cultural activities that provide them with value and an improved quality of life.

◆ Assisting a client to learn how to safely utilize public transportation to get to work if they are no longer able to drive.

◆ Guiding a client to pace daily activities to conserve energy following a concussion.

◆ Practicing with a client how to safely transfer in and out of a bathtub using a tub transfer bench and grab bars that have been installed.

♦ Assisting a client with woodworking tasks to assist with increasing their ability to return to work as a carpenter.

♦ Providing sensory integration therapy in the school system for a student with autism.

♦ Setting up a golf putting mat within a long-term care facility and assisting a resident to participate in this enjoyable leisure activity.

♦ Teaching a client with decreased upper extremity function to use an alternative communication device to assist with connecting with family, friends, and others through technology.

♦ Guiding a client in meal preparation activities in the occupational therapy department kitchen setting prior to discharge home to ensure safe operation of appliances.

Providing Client and/or Family Education

♦ Fall prevention strategies to incorporate within a client's home environment.

♦ Joint protection/energy conservation education to a client and family group.

♦ Teaching a family member how to safely assist a client to complete toilet transfers using a raised toilet seat and toilet arm rests.

♦ Reviewing wheelchair use and maintenance with a client and/or care giver.

♦ Providing processes to assist the client to problem-solve when presented with a challenging situation.

♦ Educating parents on teaching necessary skills to their child including handwriting, reading, and self-feeding.

♦ Educating a client and family member on safe transfers into and out of a vehicle following a total hip replacement surgery.

♦ Teaching a family member a specific exercise program to encourage the client to complete on a regular schedule as determined by the occupational therapist.

♦ Educating parents on exposure therapy techniques to decrease their child's anxiety.

- ◆ Teaching a client and spouse how to deal with decreased cognition in their home environment.
- ◆ Educating a family member how to re-organize a kitchen space to ensure that it is safe and efficient for the client to participate in cooking activities.
- ◆ Educating a client with rheumatoid arthritis and their partner in sexual intimacy position options to decrease pain.
- ◆ Educating a driver on correct positioning within their vehicle to provide safety and comfort while driving.
- ◆ Educating the client and family members on the correct use and care of a pressure-relieving mattress or cushion.

Interprofessional Communication

- ◆ Educating the interprofessional team on the specific tasks the OTA has been assigned for a specific client.
- ◆ Providing client updates at team meetings.
- ◆ Participating in a family meeting regarding client discharge.
- ◆ Speaking with a nurse if the client unexpectedly demonstrates decreased physical/mental or cognitive abilities to determine if the assigned occupational therapy treatment should continue.
- ◆ Participating in interprofessional communication regarding a client with another team member.
- ◆ Educating an education assistant and/or teacher within the school system on specific approaches or processes the OTA has been applying while providing assigned treatments to a student who has a sensory processing disorder. These approaches can then be used by the EA and/or teacher when working with the student.
- ◆ Participating in family and/or team meetings regarding a client with the occupational therapist present, particularly if the therapist is new or works in a casual position and is not as informed about the client as is the OTA.

Non-direct tasks include preparing materials such as client/family education resources, assembling/maintaining equipment, completing clerical tasks, and workload measurement. These non-direct tasks are often directed by the manager or other staff.

Decision to Assign Process

The 2024 WFOT *Guiding Principles for Ethical Occupational Therapy* state that "Occupational therapy tasks are assigned by occupational therapists to another person only if that individual has the required level of competency and supervision" (WFOT, 2024, p. 5). This leads to describing a process that assists occupational therapists to determine assignment and appropriate supervision of OTAs involved in occupational therapy service delivery. Many provincial regulators have created "tools" to assist in this decision making and critical thinking, and they are summarized in this section.

It is important for occupational therapists to initially consider risk factors for each potential assignment related to the following:

1. Occupational therapist competence
2. OTA(s) competence
3. Client needs and goals
4. Task(s) to be assigned
5. Environmental context

Potential risks for each of these components, as described by Gillespie (2023), are given below.

Occupational Therapist Competence

♦ Professional working relationship with the OTA(s) to whom the therapy will be assigned.
♦ The occupational therapist's ability to provide supervision as appropriate.
♦ Competence and experience in the therapy task(s) to be assigned.
♦ Adequate time available to supervise and document the process.

OTA(s) Competence

- ◆ Working relationship with the supervising occupational therapist.
- ◆ Knowledge and experience with the task(s) to be assigned.
- ◆ Judgment and ability to recognize change in client status.
- ◆ Experience anticipating needs related to a specific diagnosis.
- ◆ Their knowledge and experience within the environmental context.

Client Needs and Goals

- ◆ Stability and complexity of needs and goals (including physical, mental and social).
- ◆ Client's ability to direct care.
- ◆ Client's ability to provide informed consent.
- ◆ Client's cultural considerations.
- ◆ Client's decision-making capacity.

Task(s) to be Assigned

- ◆ Complexity of each task.
- ◆ Skills required to complete each task.
- ◆ Specific requirements of the task for the individual client.
- ◆ Need for ongoing clinical judgement by the OTA.
- ◆ Risk of harm from doing/not doing the therapy.

Environmental Context

- ◆ Availability of resources including assistive devices and finances.
- ◆ Degree of OTA independence or isolation.
- ◆ Physical barriers/hazards.
- ◆ Availability and experience with wifi/cell coverage to support supervision.
- ◆ Predictability of staffing changes in a facility or family changes within a home setting.
- ◆ Pertinent organizational policies related to the OTA performing therapy.

(Gillespie, 2023, p. 11)

After highlighting the risk factors described above, one approach would be to consider the overall degree of risk in assigning the intervention(s) by asking these two questions:

8. What would be the probability of harm to the client if the intervention(s) were assigned, or not assigned, to the OTA(s)?
9. How would the client be impacted if harm occurred?

Another option for the next step in the decision-making process is to ask the following questions that are contained within Appendix B of the Newfoundland & Labrador Occupational Therapy Board's 2021 Practice Guideline: *Task Assignment to Assistants in Occupational Therapy Service Delivery*. The structure of the questions assumes that only one OTA would be assigned the intervention/task. The occupational therapist can use the answer to each question (yes or no) to assist with making the decision to assign a task/intervention or not:

◆ Does the involvement of the OTA improve the access to quality and/or effectiveness of the occupational therapy service?
◆ Have I considered risk factors?
◆ Can I implement appropriate risk control measures?
◆ Is this task within my scope?
◆ Do I have the experience/knowledge to supervise this activity?
◆ Does the OTA have the appropriate information and training to carry out the task/intervention safely and effectively?
◆ Am I able to provide the appropriate level of supervision needed?
◆ Has the client/substitute decision maker provided informed consent to have an OTA carry out assigned occupational therapy service components?
◆ Can an appropriate supervision plan be documented?
◆ Can informed consent be documented?

♦ Can a documentation plan be outlined for the OTA?
♦ Is this a client who is receiving ongoing occupational therapy service?

(NLOTB, 2021, p. 7)

If more than one OTA would potentially be assigned the task, each OTA would need to be considered in determining the risk factors, provided with the appropriate information including a documentation plan, and be competent in the task/intervention to be assigned; finally, informed consent from the client/substitute decision maker would need to include all OTAs involved.

It is important to emphasize again the need for occupational therapists to review their provincial regulatory requirements related to assignment and supervision. For example, there may be the need to name another occupational therapist to be the secondary supervisor if the primary occupational therapist is away. This would require both occupational therapists to be competent in the assigned task and to have confidence in the competence of the OTA(s) to whom the task will be assigned.

Consultation

There is often confusion among therapists, leaders, and other healthcare professionals regarding an occupational therapist being involved in a consultation to make recommendations versus completing an assessment and assigning tasks. Consultation in occupational therapy can be described as: "The process of contributing to a client's treatment plan by providing expert advice to, offering education or training for, and/or facilitating problem-solving with another service provider or other personnel. The occupational therapist is responsible for the quality and appropriateness of the recommendations but not for the ongoing competency, behaviour, or quality of service of the other service providers or personnel" (COTBC, 2023, p. 2).

Examples of consultation could include:

♦ A private occupational therapist is asked to recommend the safest method of transferring a new resident in a long-term care facility. The transfer will be done by the resident care aides who work under the supervision of the nursing staff. The occupational therapist is accountable for the recommendations they make but this is not an assignment of task.

♦ An occupational therapist assesses a child in the school system and provides the recommended program to the teacher who supervises an education assistant. The EA would carry out the program under the supervision of the teacher.

♦ An occupational therapist recommends a home program to a client that will be delivered by a member of the client's family.

♦ An occupational therapist recommends the optimum positioning for a client in a palliative care unit.

♦ An occupational therapist recommends assistive equipment or devices for those living in a homeless shelter who have mobility issues. These recommendations can be discussed with the homeless outreach workers on the site.

♦ A client's family has hired a contractor to renovate the entrance into their home and the doorways into rooms within the home now that the family member requires a power wheelchair for mobility. The occupational therapist recommends appropriate changes to the contractor to increase accessibility for the client.

Supervision

As previously stated, the occupational therapist is responsible for supervising the OTA(s) to ensure the assigned task(s) are being delivered to the client safely and effectively. As discussed in Chapter 1, Hagler, Madill, and Kennedy (1994) stated that OTA supervision is "incumbent upon the employers, clinical administrators, program supervisors, clinical professionals, and support workers themselves to ensure that support workers do not provide occupational therapy services without supervision by an occupational therapist" (Hagler, Madill, & Kennedy, 1994, p. 216). This continues to be imperative within current clinical practice settings, and the requirement for professional development education and mentoring for therapists, practice leads, managers, and employers in the role and supervision of therapist assistants is mandatory. This will be discussed further in Chapter 5.

The occupational therapist also needs to monitor the progress of the client and modify the assigned interventions as needed. The supervision method can include a chart review as well as direct observations of the intervention delivery.

The 2019 ACOTRO position statement discusses supervision as direct, indirect, or remote.

- ◆ **Direct Supervision** – the occupational therapist is in direct visual contact with the OTA or within the vicinity.
- ◆ **Indirect Supervision** – the occupational therapist is in the same facility and can be easily contacted.
- ◆ **Remote Supervision** – the supervising occupational therapist is not on site. In this situation, there must be a plan for emergencies including a designated on-site health professional that the OTA can approach for assistance. Another option is if the supervising occupational therapist is available by teleconference (ACOTRO, 2019, pp. 2–3).

Examples of occupational therapist supervision models following assignment of tasks to OTAs in different clinical situations are discussed below.

1. An OTA within a community setting has been assigned interventions to increase food acceptance for a child with autism spectrum disorder (AHD). As this intervention often occurs in the client's home with the parents in attendance, OTA supervision by the occupational therapist would mainly be remote because the therapist and the OTA are in different locations. The occupational therapist will review the OTA's documentation following treatment sessions, and adjust the plan as needed.

The occupational therapy team in this work setting "has developed an effective process to ensure OTA implementation of individualized food acceptance programs is supervised and supported while meeting the needs of the clients and families served" (Caines, 2015, p. 7).

2. A full-time OTA who has been working in the hospital environment for one year has met a new occupational therapist recently hired full-time within the facility. The therapist had collaborated with OTAs in their previous employment and is eager to develop a therapeutic relationship with this OTA colleague. The occupational therapist has assigned the task of applying straps and monitoring the fit of a resting hand splint to the OTA for an in-patient client who recently experienced a hand injury at work. As the therapist/OTA partnership is new, the occupational therapist will initially directly supervise the OTA as they complete the assigned tasks for this client. When the therapist determines that the OTA has demonstrated the required competencies for splint completion and monitoring, the type of supervision provided for the next client assignment related to splinting would likely be indirect. However, the therapist would confirm that the OTA understood their responsibility of contacting the supervising therapist if any issues or clarification requirements surfaced during the treatment.

3. An OTA in a remote northern community who is identified as a Community Therapy Assistant (CTA) provides occupational therapy services to local clients and is supervised remotely by two occupational therapists who reside at a distance, although they do visit the community when they are able. The numerous tasks that are assigned to the CTA include "facilitating fine motor programs with children, exercise and activity re-activation programs with adults; installing assistive devices and providing training on their use; and helping maintain mobility aids" (Bellefontaine, Hurley, & Irngaut, 2015, p. 21). The CTA does communicate with the supervising therapists as

regularly as possible through telephone, email, and fax, but this can be challenging at times due to limitations in technology within the northern community. Despite these struggles, the benefits of having the CTA within their local community to enable in-person treatment sessions and to install required assistive devices "means so much to the community" (Bellefontaine, Hurley, & Irngaut, 2015, p. 22).

There is no specific ratio as to the number of OTAs that a single occupational therapist can supervise, but client safety and effectiveness of therapy delivery must always be considered (ACOTRO, 2019). The occupational therapist must be confident in the competence of each OTA included in every task assignment. As described by Blake, Park, and Brice-Leddy in their 2015 article based on a new model of care in an Ontario acute care hospital, "all assistants are required to be competent" and that "establishing a baseline competency was essential as occupational therapists are now assigning to five rotating OTA/PTAs on each unit" (Blake, Park, & Brice-Leddy, 2015, p.13). To meet this baseline competency, the article describes that a learning needs assessment was developed and distributed to the OTA/PTAs on staff, with a response rate of 100% – "a hearty indication that the OTA/PTAs were eager to address their learning needs," and a clinical learning environment was then initiated (Blake, Park, & Brice-Leddy, 2015, p. 13). This further reinforces the need for ongoing learning and professional development for OTAs; this will be reviewed in more detail in Chapter 5.

Case Studies
Case study examples including specific questions are provided to assist with the decision-making process. The answers given are from the author's perspective.

Case Study 1
Occupational Therapist and OTA Relationship
The occupational therapist has been working in home care for one year and had collaborated frequently with an OTA who

recently relocated to another city. The OTA with whom the therapist will now be working has been hired following graduation from an accredited OTA/PTA education program. The OTA had completed a fieldwork placement at another home care community setting within the same province during their education and informs the therapist that they had worked independently with a few clients during that placement.

Case Description

The occupational therapist has assessed Betty, a 70-year-old female who lives alone in a second-floor apartment with elevator access. Betty has decreased balance and ambulates with the assistance of a four-wheeled walker. Betty reports that she is afraid to shower in the bathtub as she previously experienced a fall, and as a result has only been sponge bathing to maintain cleanliness.

The occupational therapist has received permission from Betty's landlord to have grab bars installed around the bathtub, and non-slip mats both inside and outside the tub are already in place. Betty has agreed to trial a shower chair and has consented to the OTA providing therapy.

The occupational therapist is considering assigning the following task to the OTA:

◆ Practice transfers entering/exiting the bathtub using a shower chair and grab bars, and progress to improve Betty's confidence in independently showering safely.

Questions:

◆ How will the occupational therapist develop the intraprofessional relationship with the OTA?
◆ What are the risk factors for this task to be assigned?
◆ Will the occupational therapist likely assign this task? If so, what type of supervision would be provided?
◆ Is it appropriate for the OTA to select a shower chair to trial with Betty, or should the occupational therapist choose the model of shower chair for the trial?

Case Study 1 Answers

◆ **How will the occupational therapist develop the intra-professional relationship with the OTA?**

The therapist will ask the OTA more information about the therapy provided during their fieldwork placements, their understanding of cultural safety, any additional learning the OTA has achieved, their experiences with documentation, and any special interests the OTA would like to share. It would be helpful for the therapist to also understand the supervision experienced by the OTA during the home care placement and the current level of confidence the OTA has in this current community home care setting.

◆ **What are the risk factors for this task to be assigned?**

Occupational therapist competence: *Low risk*

Even though the occupational therapist has not yet worked with the OTA, the therapist has collaborated successfully with the previous OTA in the same setting.

OTA competence: *Medium risk*

The occupational therapist/OTA relationship is new, but the OTA does report having previous experience in home care during a placement in their education program.

Client needs and goals: *Low risk*

The client can direct her own care, and although Betty has a fear of showering due to a previous fall, her goal is to shower independently.

Task to be assigned: *Medium risk*

There are now grab bars installed in the bathtub along with non-slip mats in place, resulting in increased safety during Betty's transfer practice using the shower chair on trial.

Environmental context: *High risk*

The task is taking place with only Betty and the OTA in her home within the community.

◆ **Will the occupational therapist likely assign this task? If so, what type of supervision would be provided?**

The occupational therapist will assign this task with remote supervision. As this is a new collaboration, the therapist will ensure that they are available by phone if an issue occurs while the OTA is providing therapy.

◆ **Is it appropriate for the OTA to select a shower chair to trial with Betty, or should the occupational therapist choose the model of shower chair for the trial?**
As it is early in the relationship, the occupational therapist should select the shower chair to trial with the client. As their working relationship grows and the therapist is confident that the OTA could safely select an appropriate shower chair, it would be acceptable to include this option within a similar task assignment in the future.

Case Study 2
Occupational Therapist and OTA Relationship

The occupational therapist has been working in an occupational therapy private practice for two years, and the OTA has been subcontracted to the same private practice for one year and has experience working with clients experiencing mental health issues. The therapist and assistant have not previously worked together, but the occupational therapist has heard from colleagues about the successful outcomes achieved by the OTA with clients who are experiencing similar issues. The clinic's policies ensure that there is appropriate time available for therapists to supervise the OTAs as needed.

Case Description

The occupational therapist has completed an assessment with William, a 35-year-old sales manager who suffered a traumatic brain injury resulting from a motor vehicle accident. William is aware of his limitations and states that because he now becomes very anxious when surrounded by other people, there is a fear that he will not be able to return to his job or generally be engaged within society. William consents to the OTA assisting in his therapy and the therapist has confirmed with William's auto insurance provider that it will fund the OTA on the condition that the therapist provides regular updates to them.

The occupational therapist is considering assigning the following task to the OTA:

◆ Re-integrate William into community environments to decrease his anxiety of socializing and working with others, beginning with meeting a few people in controlled environments, and progressing to larger groups as appropriate.

Questions:

◆ How would the occupational therapist develop a trusting relationship with the OTA?
◆ What are the risk factors for this task to be assigned?
◆ What is the probability of harm and the impact to the client if harm occurs with each risk factor?
◆ Will the occupational therapist likely assign this intervention? If so, what type of supervision would be provided?

Case Study 2 Answers

◆ **How would the occupational therapist develop a trusting relationship with the OTA?**
The occupational therapist will initiate a conversation with the OTA to learn about their experiences with this type of therapy and working with clients experiencing anxiety following a TBI, and potentially provide learning resources on this topic. The therapist will share personal experience in this area and their expectations of the OTA regarding intraprofessional communication and documentation. The therapist could also ask the OTA to observe a therapy session with another client experiencing similar symptoms, with consent from the client.

◆ **What are the risk factors for this task to be assigned? Occupational therapist competence:** *Low risk*
The therapist has worked in the practice for two years and although the occupational therapist/OTA working relationship is new, positive feedback has been given by colleagues who have collaborated with the OTA. The clinic allows time for the required amount of supervision and documentation to occur.

OTA competence: *Low to medium risk*

Although the OTA has experience in this practice setting and providing this type of therapy for clients with similar issues, the occupational therapist/OTA working relationship is new.

Client needs and goals: *Medium risk*

William's anxiety when with other people could be a high risk, but the fact that he is aware of his limitations and able to direct his own care does decrease the risk to medium.

Task to be assigned: *Medium risk*

The task of re-integrating William into society through meeting other people could initially result in increased anxiety, and the OTA will need to provide ongoing clinical judgment.

Environmental context: *High risk*

This therapy will be provided by the OTA in the community with no other healthcare providers available for support if needed. The risk is also increased when a third-party payer is involved and this may have limitations in the amount of therapy provided.

◆ **Will the occupational therapist likely assign this task? If not, what are the reasons?**

The therapist will likely assign this task based on the OTA's experience and competence, and the fact that William is aware of his limitations due to anxiety. The therapist would specifically identify locations appropriate for the OTA to take William. Initially, they could visit a friend at their home, and then increase William's socialization by taking him to a busier environment such as a coffee shop. The grading would be determined by William's progression. The involvement of a third-party payer potentially may affect the amount of therapy the OTA is allowed to provide, which the therapist needs to understand.

◆ **If assigned, what type of supervision would the therapist provide?**

The therapist would likely provide direct supervision for the first session to observe the OTA's therapy delivery and William's interactions with the OTA. If successful, the supervision could proceed to indirect, but the therapy would only occur on days when the therapist is working to provide assistance if needed.

Case Study 3
Occupational Therapist and OTA Relationship

The occupational therapist has worked three days/week in a rural community practice for one year. There is a part-time physiotherapist on staff, and a full-time OTA/PTA has recently been hired. The OTA/PTA has five years' experience in a rural hospital following graduation from an accredited education program and has worked under the supervision of both an occupational therapist and a physiotherapist. The OTA/PTA mainly treated adult clients experiencing a broad range of physical and cognitive limitations.

Case Description

Savannah has been referred to physiotherapy and occupational therapy at the community clinic following a recent fall resulting in a right shoulder injury. She did not require surgery and is right hand dominant. A year ago, she had been diagnosed with early-stage vascular dementia. She lives with her older husband in a one-level home.

The physiotherapist has assigned the OTA/PTA a daily exercise program to complete with Savannah at her home.

The occupational therapist is considering assigning the following task to the OTA:

- ◆ Food preparation activities to increase Savannah's independence and safety in providing meals for herself and her husband, beginning with simple cooking activities and progressing to more challenging tasks as appropriate.
- ◆ The OTA/PTA will visit Savannah at her home to complete this activity in addition to the exercise program assigned by the physiotherapist.

Questions

- ◆ What does the OTA/PTA need to understand about the task assignments by the physiotherapist and the occupational therapist?
- ◆ How should the OTA/PTA approach Savannah regarding the choice of meal activity to be completed?

◆ How does the OTA/PTA respond if an issue arises with Savannah while performing the meal preparation activity on a day when the occupational therapist is not working but the physiotherapist is working?

◆ What would be the best way for the occupational therapist to evaluate the result of this task assignment?

Case Study 3 Answers

◆ **What does the OTA/PTA need to understand about the task assignments by the physiotherapist and the occupational therapist?**

As the physiotherapist is responsible for treatment they have assigned and the occupational therapist is responsible for the treatment they have assigned, the OTA/PTA needs to understand that if any issues arise while delivering the exercise program, the physiotherapist needs to be contacted, and if any concerns arise while doing meal preparation, the occupational therapist needs to be contacted.

◆ **How should the OTA/PTA approach Savannah regarding the choice of meal activity to be completed?**

The OTA/PTA needs to discuss options of meals with Savannah, in particular the time required to complete the cooking activity, ensuring it is within the treatment schedule and within any boundaries set by the occupational therapist in the supervision plan, to understand any cultural considerations and ask Savannah about this if needed, and to check that all required items are available. Due to Savannah's early-stage vascular dementia, the OTA/PTA should also consider a familiar meal prep activity that is not too complicated for Savannah to complete. They will decide on a chosen activity together.

◆ **How does the OTA/PTA respond if an issue arises with Savannah while performing the meal preparation activity on a day when the occupational therapist is not working but the physiotherapist is working?**

The OTA/PTA can contact the physiotherapist if an issue arises while performing meal preparation (as they are familiar with

Savannah), and the physiotherapist can provide recommendations as to how to approach the issue or recommend that the OTA/PTA discontinue the treatment if necessary. However, as the occupational therapist is the supervising therapist, the OTA/PTA (and the physiotherapist) will document the issue within Savannah's health record BUT they must inform the occupational therapist once back at work. The occupational therapist will then reassess Savannah and potentially change the treatment program.

♦ **What would be the best way for the occupational therapist to evaluate the result of this task assignment?**

The occupational therapist will reassess Savannah's meal preparation abilities following treatment to determine if her status has improved, and specifically ask Savannah how she feels about her ability to prepare meals, and her opinions on working with the OTA/PTA. The occupational therapist will also discuss the process with the OTA/PTA as to successes and/or issues experienced during the treatment.

Case Study 4
Occupational Therapist and OTA Relationship

The occupational therapist has worked at a private clinic for three months and has successfully assigned low-risk tasks to the OTA on the staff who has worked at the clinic for one year. The outcomes of the OTA treatments assigned by the occupational therapist to date have assisted the clients in reaching their goals. A new referral has been received for client John, who has been diagnosed with multiple sclerosis resulting in decreased mobility. John is requesting a power wheelchair and informs the occupational therapist that funding should be available from his provincial benefits plan.

Case Description

The occupational therapist has assessed John and has determined that a power wheelchair trial is appropriate to determine John's safe ability to operate the device within his community. John demonstrates adequate functional cognition, and lives alone in an accessible condominium complex. His main occupational therapy goal is to remain independent with mobility access for as long as possible.

The occupational therapist has completed power mobility trials in past experiences but has not assigned this intervention previously to an OTA. However, it has been confirmed that the OTA has already been assigned this task by another occupational therapist at the clinic.

The occupational therapist is considering assigning the following task to the OTA:

♦ A power wheelchair trial in collaboration with a local medical vendor to determine if John can safely operate the appropriate power wheelchair within his community. The distance from John's home to each trial's destination will progress as John's ability to operate the power wheelchair improves.

Questions

♦ What are the risk factors for assigning this task?
♦ How would the occupational therapist determine the OTA's competence in performing this task?
♦ As funding for the power wheelchair may be available from a provincial benefits plan, what information does the occupational therapist need to be aware of if the power mobility practice is assigned to the OTA?
♦ If the occupational therapist decides to assign this task to the OTA, what type of supervision would be appropriate to include in the supervision plan?

Case Study 4 Answers

♦ **What are the risk factors for assigning this task?**
  Occupational therapist competence: *Low risk*
  The occupational therapist has completed power mobility trials with previous clients and is competent with this process. Although the therapist has not assigned this intervention to

the OTA, the tasks previously assigned have been successful although they were considered lower risk.

OTA competence: *Low risk*

The OTA has been assigned this task by another occupational therapist in the same clinic and is familiar with this intervention.

Client needs and goals: *Medium risk*

John has multiple sclerosis which is a progressive disease, and their ability may decline during the power mobility trial. However, John's goal is to remain independent as long as possible which increases motivation.

Task to be assigned: *High risk*

Operating a power wheelchair device within a community is high risk due to the need to safely cross busy roads and the power wheelchair may not be seen by motorists.

Environmental context: *High risk*

The OTA will be performing this task alone with the client in a community setting.

◆ **How would the occupational therapist determine the OTA's competence in performing this task?**

The occupational therapist could discuss the OTA's competence with their occupational therapist colleague who had previously assigned power mobility practice to the OTA. However, even with this conversation occurring, the occupational therapist would still need to observe the OTA performing this task at least once to determine competence. Based on the result, the therapist would then determine whether to assign or not.

◆ **As funding for the power wheelchair may be available from a provincial benefits plan, what information does the occupational therapist need to be aware of if the power mobility practice is assigned to the OTA?**

As each funding agency has different requirements within their funding processes, the occupational therapist would need confirmation from the funder that the OTA can perform this power mobility task. If so, the occupational therapist would need to obtain consent from the client for the OTA to be involved in this intervention and confirm with the funder if verbal consent is sufficient or if written consent is required.

◆ **If the occupational therapist decides to assign this task to the OTA, what type of supervision would be appropriate to include in the supervision plan?**
As there is high risk involved in this assignment, the supervision would initially be direct and the occupational therapist would observe at least one power mobility practice session. If this is successful, the supervision could be indirect, but the intervention would only be performed on days the occupational therapist is working at the clinic. If the therapist called in sick on a day that a training session with the client was planned, the OTA would need to reschedule the appointment.

Case Study 5
Occupational Therapist and OTA Relationship
The occupational therapist has been working in the public school system for five years and has assigned tasks to other OTAs within the system. They are introduced to a newly hired OTA who recently graduated from an accredited program. Prior to entering the therapist assistant education program, the OTA was employed as an educational assistant (EA) in another school system within the area.

Case Description
The occupational therapist has assessed Miki, a six-year-old student, who has demonstrated decreased fine motor skill development which is contributing to difficulty with printing in school. Following the assessment and discussion with Miki's parents as to the recommended treatment plan, they have consented to have the OTA involved in Miki's therapy. The task assignment is to improve ability and confidence to print, enabling Miki to better participate in school learning activities.

The occupational therapist is considering assigning the following task to the OTA:

◆ Practice fine motor skill development and improve Miki's ability to print. This would assist Miki to improve his confidence in printing, enabling him to better participate in school learning.

Questions

♦ Does the occupational therapist need to discuss with the OTA their previous role as an EA as they develop their therapeutic working relationship? If so, what factors does the OTA need to be aware of?
♦ What are the risk factors related to this assignment?
♦ Would the occupational therapist likely assign this task based on risk factors?
♦ If Miki's parents asked the OTA about Miki's progress with printing skills, how would the OTA respond?

Case Study 5 Answers

♦ **Does the occupational therapist need to discuss with the OTA their previous role as an EA as they develop their therapeutic working relationship? If so, what factors does the OTA need to be aware of?**
Yes, the occupational therapist needs to ensure the OTA understands that direction/supervision is given by the occupational therapist, not the teacher as would have been the case in the OTA's previous role as an EA. In addition, the OTA needs to know that tasks assigned are directed by the occupational therapist. The teacher should also understand this process.

♦ **What are the risk factors related to this assignment?**
Occupational therapist competence: *Low risk*
The occupational therapist has worked in the system for five years and assigned tasks to other OTAs.
OTA competence: *High risk*
The OTA is new to this school system and a recent graduate of an education program. If the OTA had experienced a similar task assignment during a fieldwork placement the risk would potentially be lowered. If the OTA had performed a task related to this assignment when they worked as an EA the risk also could be potentially lowered – although it could also increase the risk depending on how they had been instructed to teach a student this task.

Client needs and goals: *Low risk*
Miki is demonstrating decreased fine motor skills but is otherwise healthy.
Task to be assigned: *Low risk*
Improving Miki's ability and confidence in printing is a low-risk task.
Environmental context: *Low risk*
The public school system is a safe environment.

◆ **Would the occupational therapist likely assign this task based on risk factors?**
Yes, the occupational therapist would likely assign this task even though their relationship with the OTA is in the early stages of development. The occupational therapist's competence, the client's needs and goals, the intervention, and the environment are all low risk.

◆ **If Miki's parents asked the OTA about Miki's progress with printing skills, how would the OTA respond?**
The OTA would respond that the occupational therapist will need to be informed of their question as it is not within the OTA's role to report on a client's progress. The OTA could inform the parents that they will pass this question on to the supervising occupational therapist.

Supervision and Communication Plan

If an occupational therapist decides to assign a task (or intervention) to an OTA, the next step is to develop and document a supervision and communication plan as required by many of the regulation documents. The components of the supervision plan must include the following:

◆ The specific task(s) assigned with instructions or reference to a care protocol. This would include the extent to which the task(s) can be progressed.
◆ Name and title of the OTA or a specific roster of OTAs if all are competent in the task.

- ◆ Frequency of OTA intervention.
- ◆ Documentation that informed consent was obtained from the client or substitute decision maker (SDM) for OTA involvement in the occupational therapy service delivery.
- ◆ Type of supervision that will be provided by the supervising occupational therapist including direct, indirect, or remote.
- ◆ Method and frequency of communication between the OTA(s) and the supervising occupational therapist.

If provincial regulations require that a secondary occupational therapist be identified if the supervising occupational therapist is unavailable, the name of the secondary occupational therapist would need to be given in the supervision plan.

Supervision Plan Examples

Examples of occupational therapists' documented supervision plans for specific case studies have been provided below, based on the author's knowledge and experience.

Case Example 1

John is a 59-year-old male who recently suffered a right CVA and has been admitted to the hospital acute care unit. His perceptual abilities have remained functional and his physical limitations are slight weakness in his left upper and lower extremities, but his main deficit is cognitive impairment. He works as an accountant and is anxious to return to work. During the initial assessment, his behavior demonstrates frustration with his current limitations, and he is easily distracted.

There are two OTAs on the neurological unit, Mary and Jane. As an occupational therapist, you have worked with both of them for the past six months and a trusting professional working relationship has been developed. You have decided to assign cognitive retraining activities to the OTAs with the client's consent.

Documented Supervision Plan

Following informed consent from client John, cognitive retraining tasks have been assigned to OTA Mary and OTA Jane to be completed once daily in a one-to-one treatment session. The cognitive skills to be included are short-term memory, attention, and problem-solving as documented in the client record. As John is currently easily distracted, the initial treatment sessions are to be a maximum of 30 minutes, grading the time frame based on his performance and behavior. Document within the health record following each client interaction and report to supervising occupational therapist a minimum of twice weekly in person or via cell phone. The supervision will be indirect. If a concern arises and the occupational therapist is not available, the OTA working with John is to report to the therapy manager to determine appropriate action. John will be reassessed in one week or earlier if his status changes.

This supervision plan may change based on new factors that occur. For example, if OTA Mary informs the occupational therapist that while she was working with John earlier in the day, his frustration increases to a much higher level, the therapist may need to provide direct supervision during the following session to observe his behavior and possibly reconsider this assignment of task.

Case Example 2

Bill is a 75-year-old gentleman who has been developing weakness in his lower extremities which is affecting his longer distance mobility. He lives alone in a main-level condominium and needs to access the grocery store located in his neighborhood. The occupational therapist working in community care determines that a trial of a power wheelchair would be appropriate to determine his ability to safely mobilize based on her initial assessment of Bill.

A new OTA, Phil, has been recently hired within the organization, and he has previous experience working in the local hospital. In your capacity as an occupational therapist, you have been working with Phil for the past two weeks, and this is the first power wheelchair trial in which Phil will be involved under your supervision. You decide to assign power mobility practice to Phil to work along with the medical vendor who will bring the power wheelchair to Bill's home for trial.

Documented Supervision Plan

Informed consent was received from client Bill to proceed with a power wheelchair trial as recommended following the occupational therapy assessment, and Bill agreed to work with OTA Phil for power wheelchair training. Jack, who works with medical vendor ABC will provide the power wheelchair for each session. OTA Phil will practice with Bill twice a week for two weeks to safely exit and re-enter his condo building via the doorways and elevator and then proceed to the grocery store one block away when OTA Phil, in discussion with the supervising occupational therapist, determines it is safe to do so. Occupational therapist supervision will be direct for the initial two visits and move to remote supervision for remaining visits if appropriate. OTA Phil will complete the Power Mobility Checklist and will document following each visit. A reassessment by this occupational therapist will be scheduled with Bill in two weeks.

Case Example 3

Paul is experiencing depression following the tragic loss of his partner from a motor vehicle accident. He now lives alone, and he had to take a leave of absence from his job in the retail sector due to his lack of motivation affecting his occupational participation. Paul has started attending an out-patient clinic in a mental health setting three times per week and has been assessed by the contracted occupational therapist. During the assessment, Paul states that one activity he previously enjoyed was photography but he has not participated in this occupation since his loss.

OTA Marie, who worked in an orthopedic clinic prior to being hired at the facility, has completed a professional development education module to better understand mental health conditions including how to approach and work with clients based on their symptoms. Marie has also collaborated with the occupational therapist in the provision of various treatments as a further learning tool.

Following the assessment, the occupational therapist has decided to assign the activity of photography to OTA Marie to help motivate Paul to return to an occupation he previously enjoyed.

Documented Supervision Plan

Informed consent has been provided by Paul to have OTA Marie assist in increasing Paul's participation within the activity of photography. This therapy will occur on Monday, Wednesday, and Friday initially for 30 minutes and increase to 60 minutes based on Paul's tolerance, for the next three weeks. OTA Marie will initiate the treatment by taking Paul outdoors and encourage him to take photos of scenes that interest him and encourage communication throughout each session including his review of the photos he has taken. The length of each session will be increased as appropriate. This occupational therapist will provide direct supervision for the initial two sessions to ensure OTA Marie's competence in this assignment and will indirectly supervise for the remaining sessions. OTA Marie is to contact the supervising occupational therapist by cell phone if an issue arises and will approach the clinic nurse if urgent attention is needed and the therapist is unavailable. OTA Marie is to document in Paul's chart following each session and an occupational therapist reassessment will be scheduled in three weeks.

Case Example 4

The occupational therapist is employed part-time at an assisted living facility along with a part-time physical therapist and two full-time OTA/PTAs, one having been recently hired. The occupational therapist has worked with OTA/PTA Kim but has yet to develop a working relationship with OTA/PTA Matt.

Albert, aged 82, has recently moved into the assisted living facility following a CVA resulting in right hemiparesis in upper and lower extremities, and is experiencing difficulties feeding himself. Albert was living at home alone prior to the onset of the CVA and did not feel safe returning to that environment. Following the occupational therapist's assessment, one of the occupational performance goals established by the therapist and the client is to increase independence and safety with feeding tasks. The occupational therapist has decided to assign the task of assisting Albert to feed himself safely utilizing appropriate assistive devices to OTA Kim.

Documented Supervision Plan

Informed consent was obtained from client Albert for OTA Kim to be involved in feeding activities. OTA Kim will teach Albert to use appropriate assistive devices to compensate for limitations as described by this occupational therapist, during breakfast and lunch each day for five days, and will document in Albert's chart once daily. Occupational therapist supervision will be indirect or remote depending on the day, and OTA Kim will approach the facility nursing supervisor if an issue arises and the supervising occupational therapist is not available. An occupational therapist reassessment with Albert will be scheduled in one week.

It is important for OTA Matt to understand that this intervention has not been assigned to him, and that if OTA Kim was absent on a day that the occupational therapist was not working, Matt could not be involved in assisting Albert with feeding as this treatment was not assigned to him. It is beneficial if the interprofessional team members also have this understanding and do not pressure Matt to assist with Albert's feeding, as this would place Matt in an uncomfortable situation.

Case Example 5

You are a new occupational therapist on an orthopedic unit in an acute care hospital and have had minimal experience working with therapist assistants. As part of your orientation, you were required to complete an online education course on supervising OTAs and needed to take the time to develop working relationships with the three OTA/PTAs who regularly work on the orthopedic unit.

Yan, a 70-year-old widow, had a right total hip arthroplasty two days ago due to progressive osteoarthritis. She lives alone in a one-level home and is looking forward to returning home. She is currently ambulating safely with a two-wheeled walker. Following your occupational therapy initial assessment, you have decided to assign the interventions of practicing lower limb dressing and toilet/tub transfers to the OTA/PTAs on the unit.

Documented Supervision Plan

Informed consent was received from the client to assign lower extremity dressing practice and toilet/bathtub transfers to the ortho unit OTA/PTAs, as outlined in the client's occupational therapy plan. The involved OTA/PTA will document the daily participation and progress of the client, and the supervising occupational therapist will review documentation in preparation for discharge planning. Supervision will be indirect, and OTAs can contact this occupational therapist by cell phone if an issue arises.

If the supervising occupational therapist is confident in the competence of each OTA/PTA working in a specific area, tasks can be assigned to the OTA/PTAs as a group, in this case the "ortho unit OTA/PTAs," with each person's name listed on a roster within the unit. If a casual OTA/PTA or new OTA/PTA was working on a particular day, they could not be included in the assignment until their name was added to the roster.

Case Example 6

You are an occupational therapist located in a community center that serves a remote community and have worked one year with OTA Josee who is a graduate from an accredited OTA/PTA education program.

Randall is 52 years old and recently suffered a fractured pelvis from a fall on the ice. He lives with his wife in a one-level home and was discharged from hospital yesterday. You completed your occupational therapy assessment virtually as Randall lives a long distance away, and Randall's primary goal is to shower independently in his bathtub. You have assigned OTA Josee, who lives closer to Randall, to determine whether a transfer tub bench will fit in his bathroom and, if so, to practice transfers with Randall and decide if he is safe to complete his showering tasks independently.

Documented Supervision Plan

Informed consent was received from the client Randall during the virtual occupational therapy assessment for OTA Josee to visit Randall at his home to trial a transfer tub bench in his bathroom. If OTA Josee determines that the bench fits safely, practicing transferring on/off the bench followed by shower practice will proceed. Josee OTA will then revisit the client within a week to ensure that the transfer and showering is safe and the client is satisfied. If the bench does not fit safely, OTA Josee will contact this occupational therapist to discuss further shower bench options. OTA Josee will document in the client's chart following each visit and will contact the supervising occupational therapist by cell phone if questions arise. The occupational therapist will supervise remotely. An occupational therapy reassessment will be completed virtually once the appropriate equipment device is in place.

OTA Documentation

OTA responsibilities for documentation, or record keeping, vary across practice areas, employer organizations, and provinces/ territories. It is critical that OTAs learn the required method of documentation within each clinical practice area where they are treating clients, and also find out if each specific supervising therapist has any particular requirements for the OTA to include within their client documentation.

The CAOT *Competencies for Occupational Therapist Assistants* state in Domain B, *Communication and Collaboration*, that:

> **The competent OTA is expected to:**
> ◆ **B2 Maintain professional documentation**
>   • **B2.1** Maintain clear, accurate, and timely records following all applicable provincial, regulatory, and organizational standards.
>   • **B2.2** Maintain confidentiality, security, and data integrity in the sharing, transmission, storage, and management of information.
>   • **B2.3** Use electronic and digital technologies responsibly.
>
> (CAOT, 2024, p. 8)

The occupational therapist is responsible for ensuring that appropriate records are kept related to assignment of tasks to

OTAs (ACOTRO, 2019). Based on the communication and direction by the supervising occupational therapist, the OTAs will record assigned interventions on the client record as required. They must make sure that they are meeting the above competency requirements. The OTA must sign the documentation using their appropriate title. Co-signing the OTA documentation by the supervising therapist may be required by a facility or organization but is not a consistent requirement (ACOTRO, 2019).

Professional Liability Insurance

A topic that needs to be discussed at this point is professional liability insurance for OTA/PTAs working in Canada. Many healthcare employers do provide professional liability insurance for therapists and therapist assistants, but the terms are often misunderstood. Therefore, it is important that all employees, including occupational therapists and OTAs, understand the limits and restrictions that may affect them individually.

It has also been noted that certain employers across the country are no longer providing liability insurance, resulting in each employee being responsible for purchasing their own insurance.

Professional liability insurance can be purchased by members of the Canadian Physiotherapy Association (CPA) or the Canadian Association of Occupational Therapists (CAOT). OTAs and PTAs who meet the membership criteria can purchase this insurance through either the CPA or the CAOT, and the combined insurance protects them when working as an OTA under the supervision of an occupational therapist and/or as a PTA under the supervision of a physiotherapist.

This multi-disciplinary coverage protects OTAs and/or PTAs against liability, or allegations of liability, from injury or damages to a client, or potential other third party. This injury or damage could result from an error, omission, negligent act, or malpractice that has arisen out of the professional capacity of an OTA and/or a PTA (CAOT, 2022–23; CPA, 2023–24).

Examples of situations when an OTA may require professional liability insurance could include:

- ◆ Client alleges that misinformation was provided by the OTA regarding the assigned treatment.
- ◆ An error was made during the delivery of occupational therapy treatment by the OTA.
- ◆ The OTA has gone beyond the assigned treatment limitations documented by the occupational therapist within the supervision plan and the client experiences an injury.
- ◆ Client alleges that the OTA breached their confidentiality by sharing their personal information.
- ◆ The OTA's documentation was not as transparent and detailed as required, resulting in a lack of clarity as to the treatment that was provided.
- ◆ An OTA provided occupational therapy treatment to a client that was not assigned to them by an occupational therapist.

It is strongly recommended that OTAs find out if professional liability insurance is available for them through their employer and, if so, understand the limitations of the insurance related to certain situations. Based on their findings, it would be beneficial to explore other available options prior to a situation occurring where having the insurance would be valuable.

Review Questions

To reinforce a clear understanding of terms and processes within this chapter, review questions are listed below that could be applied to employee or contracted positions within occupational therapy. It is recommended that these questions be considered according to the reader's current or future role as it relates to occupational therapy – this can include a clinical occupational therapist, student occupational therapist, rehabilitation practice leader, manager of occupational therapy staff, OTA, student OTA, occupational therapist educator, and OTA educator.

1. Explain the difference between assignment and delegation as it applies to OTAs.
2. Does an occupational therapist assign treatments to an OTA when consulting with a client? Explain why or why not.
3. What resources would contribute to an occupational therapist's decision-making process of whether to assign to an OTA or not based on provincial/territorial location?
4. Describe the limitations of OTAs within the interprofessional team.
5. What are the required components of a supervision plan?

Frequently Asked Questions

1. **Are OTAs able to develop education resources for clients?**

   Yes, *OTAs* can create education resources for clients, family members, and caregivers. The development of these resources can be assigned by the supervising occupational therapist or the practice leader, and could also involve a collaboration with another team member who contributes appropriate information if this is suitable for the particular situation. The resources can be in a written format, a pamphlet, an online resource, or any other option that is suitable for the potential users.

   OTA *graduates* from accredited education programs are familiar with researching resources to validate specific information while completing course-required assignments and projects. This is also an activity that often occurs during fieldwork placement experiences, to assist the OTA student to become more knowledgeable about particular medical conditions or to increase their understanding of a specific treatment.

2. Can OTAs teach tasks to healthcare aides?

If the *supervising* occupational therapist has directed the OTA to review specific tasks to the appropriate healthcare aides or personal care workers who will be assisting their client in care, this teaching by the OTA can be completed as documented. It would be beneficial if the supervisor of the healthcare aides (often a nurse) could be present for this teaching to ensure that there is consistency within the team. *Examples* of these tasks could include the following:

◆ Teaching about the safest and most effective method of transferring a client from their wheelchair to their hospital bed.

◆ Demonstrating how to confirm that the correct amount of air is within an air cushion (such as a ROHO cushion) positioned on the client's wheelchair to ensure optimal skin protection and prevent pressure ulcers. Additionally, reinforcing that no additional coverings such as incontinent pads are placed on the air cushion, as this will decrease the protection provided by the cushion.

◆ Reinforcing the importance of recognizing a client's specific needs related to their culture when providing care in the client's home, needs which have been learned by the OTA while they have worked with the client and their family.

◆ Educating the care workers on the safest method to assist with showering a client in their home bathroom utilizing a shower chair, grab bars, and ensuring non-slip mats are in place.

◆ Explaining the most effective use of adapted utensils to assist a resident within a long-term care facility to feed themselves safely.

◆ Instructing a healthcare aide in the optimal position for a child to be placed within their hospital bed based on a specific injury they have experienced.

◆ Providing suggestions as to decreasing a client's anxiety within a mental health facility by speaking calmly and respecting psychological safety for the client.

◆ Educating the care aides on the need for specific wheelchair adjustments and positioning of particular parts to ensure that the client is safely supported.

◆ Teaching care aides how to don and doff a client's compression stockings as long as the nursing staff agree with the specific technique used by the OTA.

◆ Providing suggestions to the care aides on communication strategies to use with a resident in their care facility, particularly regarding those residents with advancing dementia. Correcting what a resident has said will likely increase their agitation. Regardless of accuracy, it is better to agree with the resident or communicate information about the topic that will be calming, and then redirect the resident to an activity they enjoy.

3. **What leisure activities can an OTA lead in a long-term care facility?**

OTAs can *lead* numerous types of leisure activities within long-term care facilities as assigned by the supervising occupational therapist, based on the resources being available and the activities being safe for each involved resident to perform. An important consideration for the supervising occupational therapist and the OTA to understand when deciding on specific activities is that each individual resident needs to be interested in participating in the specific leisure activity that is being offered. It cannot be assumed that every resident would want to do each activity. An example where this could be a problem is asking a particular resident to participate in a cooking group within the therapeutic kitchen area of the care facility. This resident does not want to be involved in this activity as they completed cooking tasks throughout their adult life to feed their family and no longer have any interest in cooking. However, they are afraid that if they do not participate, it may cause a problem with the OTA.

The *discussion* on interested leisure activities can initially be discussed with the resident and/or family members to introduce options. A specific activity can then be trialed with the resident, with appropriate adaptations included based on the resident's abilities and limitations. Examples of activities that could be provided by the OTA include:

- ◆ Participating in simple gardening tasks outdoors including planting flowers, weeding, and/or watering the plants.
- ◆ Practicing putting a golf ball on a golf putting mat.
- ◆ Painting or drawing a picture of their favorite scenery.
- ◆ Putting together a collage of pictures from magazines based on a similar theme.
- ◆ Knitting or crocheting simple projects.
- ◆ Planning a "coffee and conversation" group to discuss current events. The invitation can be put out to a group of residents and they can choose to join or not. Coffee will be provided by the facility staff, and the OTA could potentially review the local newspaper to initiate certain discussions, and ask the residents for their views, experiences, and interest regarding specific topics.
- ◆ Leading a singing group and encouraging the residents to participate if they know the words to the songs.
- ◆ Playing board games that can be completed within a reasonable time frame.
- ◆ Putting together a jigsaw puzzle that is not too difficult or large to complete.

4. **Can occupational therapists assign treatments to kinesiologists, education assistants, and driver instructors (in Driver Rehab Programs)?**

Yes, *occupational* therapists can assign treatments to those in the above question for delivery to specific clients. It is important to note that the same process for assigning will apply to this group as it does to assigning to OTAs, and that the occupational therapist is responsible for supervising the kinesiologist, education assistant, or driver instructor when a task has been assigned to them. It must be reinforced here that if a member of this group is working with the same client providing treatment that has not been assigned by the occupational therapist, it is not considered to be occupational therapy treatment. Examples could include:

◆ A kinesiologist who works in a private clinic is visiting a client in their home to lead them in an exercise program for strengthening their upper extremity muscles following an injury. They will also instruct the client in how to dress themselves safely and independently and in the use of assistive devices if required. The dressing practice was assigned by the occupational therapist who will remotely supervise the kinesiologist as they follow the assignment protocols. The exercise program will be planned and completed by the kinesiologist based on their professional knowledge and skills, and therefore there will be no supervision for this component of the treatment.

◆ An occupational therapist working in the school system has assigned to the education assistant (EA) the task of ensuring proper positioning for a student in their wheelchair while working at their desk. The teacher has asked the education assistant to assist the student with specific reading tasks. The occupational therapist will supervise the education assistant (directly, indirectly, or remotely according to where the occupational therapist is located on that day) in adjusting the wheelchair positioning as required. The teacher will monitor the education assistant's work with the student's reading activities.

◆ An occupational therapist is involved in driver rehabilitation with a client who has specific needs related to a previous injury. The occupational therapist will assign and appropriately supervise specific requirements that the certified driver instructor needs to incorporate within their teaching to meet the client's needs. These could include proper positioning in the vehicle, appropriate communication strategies during verbal instruction, and transfers into and out of the vehicle including access and storage of required mobility devices. The driving instruction is completed by the driving instructor and is not supervised by the occupational therapist.

It is imperative that everyone involved in these situations understands the role of assignment and supervision by the occupational therapist to ensure optimal client safety. This includes the client, the kinesiologist, education assistant, or driver instructor and their managers and employers.

5. **Is it appropriate for an occupational therapist to assign an OTA to complete a cognitive screen with a client?**
   The assignment of administering cognitive assessment screens has been a frequent topic of discussion over recent years and is becoming more common in practice. This also applies to other assessment screens including the Berg Balance Scale and the Timed Up and Go tests which are often assigned by physiotherapists to PTAs but can also be assigned by occupational therapists to OTAs. Within occupational therapy, the assignment of completing screening tests, including the cognitive assessments, is considered by some therapists to be a role-emerging OTA practice component and others have been assigning this task regularly throughout a longer period of time. It is dependent on each client situation as to whether the task of administering a cognitive screen should be assigned to OTAs. As previously discussed, it is based on the factors involved in the decision to assign process and the level of risk that could be involved. There are various cognitive screens that could be applicable to this category including the MMSE, MoCA (training and certification is required), Cognistat, and SLUMS. It would be appropriate to assign to an OTA competent in this task in the following case study situation:
   ♦ The OTA has been assigned cognitive retraining treatment to a client who suffered a concussion following a

motor vehicle accident. During the initial assessment, the occupational therapist administered a standardized cognitive screen with the results indicating moderate cognitive impairment. The OTA has observed improvements in the client's cognitive performance following two weeks of cognitive retraining tasks. The occupational therapist could ask the OTA to administer the same cognitive screen used in the initial assessment (again, depending on the OTA's competence with administering this screening tool) to determine if there has been an objective improvement in the client's cognition based on the test score. The OTA would not interpret the results from the cognitive screen as this would be done by the occupational therapist. This could be an appropriate assignment with this client.

The assignment of administering a standardized cognitive screen to an OTA would not be appropriate if contributing to the discharge planning of the client or if the risk of this assignment was high.

6. **If an occupational therapist is hired in a casual position, can they assign tasks to an OTA?**
The initial response to this question is "it depends." If the occupational therapist is working consistent shifts over a period of time, is able to supervise appropriately, and has developed effective relationships with the OTAs, they will likely be able to assign treatments. If the therapist works for a few days at a time or for one week each month, they likely would not assign treatments to OTAs as they would not be able to supervise as needed throughout the extent of the therapy. However, if the therapy was short-term, for example if the therapist fabricated a splint and needed the OTA to apply straps and smooth the edges of the splint, this task could be assigned as long as the therapist is aware of the competency skills of the participating OTA. This is another illustration that demonstrates that each treatment situation is unique as to whether tasks can be assigned.

7. **If an OTA is hired in a casual position, can occupational therapists assign tasks to them?**

As in the previous question, the first reply is "it depends." If the occupational therapist assigning treatment has confidence in the casual OTA's competence in the skills required to perform the specific treatment and in addition they have developed a positive collaborative relationship, the therapist could proceed with assigning to the OTA. If the OTA's work schedule is limited due to their casual employment status, the occupational therapist would need to include other OTAs in the assignment if they are available. Additionally, this would be based on each OTA's skillset and the relationship between the therapist and the individual OTA. It is also important to note that if an OTA misses a work shift due to illness or another personal issue, the OTAs who can proceed with a client's treatment are only those that have been named in the documented supervision plan, which could also include OTAs hired in casual positions. An exception to this would be if the supervising therapist decided to update the supervision plan to include additional OTAs when informed that the OTA assigned to perform the task would not be working that day. It is important to clarify in this situation that a leader or manager within the organization cannot direct an OTA to treat a client if the OTA is not included within the documentation as this is the supervising occupational therapist's responsibility.

8. **Can an OTA work on a weekend when no occupational therapist is working?**

OTAs can work on weekends BUT the occupational therapist who has assigned the treatment remains the supervisor from a remote perspective, even though the therapist is not working during this time frame. The OTA cannot be supervised by other team members or healthcare professionals, and this includes nurses, physiotherapists, and others. However, if an urgent issue arises with a client and the OTA requires assistance or guidance, they can request help from an available healthcare professional within the setting. The healthcare professional who provides the needed care and assistance is clearly responsible for the treatment they provide in emergency situations, but the supervising occupational therapist remains responsible for the overall assigned treatment even when they are not working. This responsibility includes completing a review of the situation within the client's health record and communicating with the OTA and other involved personnel regarding the situation upon their return to work.

9. **Is it appropriate for OTAs to provide occupational therapy services when the only occupational therapist within the work setting has resigned and the position is vacant?**

   No, an OTA cannot continue to provide occupational therapy treatments if the supervising occupational therapist is no longer working in their clinical role within the work setting. An OTA can only provide occupational therapy treatments if assigned by an employed or contracted occupational therapist who is also available to supervise directly, indirectly, or remotely. However, if the OTA is also educated and trained as a PTA and there is a physiotherapist available within the work setting, they can provide assigned physiotherapy treatments to clients under the supervision of the physiotherapist.

10. **If an OTA is unable to complete an assigned treatment to a client due to time restrictions, how is this dealt with?**

    The OTA must report this to the supervising occupational therapist as soon as possible and the therapist can then determine if the treatment and/or the schedule can potentially be modified. The occupational therapist may also want to observe the OTA delivering the assigned treatment and possibly offer alternate methods or processes to use that could be more time efficient. As a result of the OTA reporting this issue right away, the client's treatment progression should not be impacted. The OTA must feel comfortable about reporting this to the supervising occupational therapist, further emphasizing the importance of developing the occupational therapist and

OTA therapeutic working relationship to ensure that the client receives the ultimate therapy service delivery.

11. **Why would I assign treatment to an OTA when the reason I became an occupational therapist is to help clients improve?**

This question has often been asked by student occupational therapists and recent occupational therapist graduates. As it is necessary for an occupational therapist to demonstrate competence in the required skills to treat their client population, they will need to follow through on treatments when beginning their career and possibly when starting a new job within an unfamiliar work setting. However, once the therapist is aware of the skills required to provide the treatments to the clients in their work setting, they should assign these to OTAs with whom they have developed therapeutic relationships and whom they are able to supervise. The fact that OTAs are educated and trained to provide client treatments provides the therapist with increased opportunities to assess for and address more occupational therapy needs for a larger number of clients in a timely and effective manner.

12. **How does an OTA/PTA prioritize assigned treatments between physiotherapy and occupational therapy?**

Conversations over the years have revealed that in many clinical work situations, the PTA role is emphasized more than the OTA role, resulting in challenges for OTAs and PTAs to decide on prioritizing client treatment assignments. Discussed already in Chapter 2, this emphasizes the importance of developing positive interprofessional relationships including understanding each other's communication needs or emotional magnets, as described by Sandy Gerber (Gerber, 2022). An effective collaboration process to assist OTAs and PTAs in determining their daily work schedule is for the occupational therapist and physiotherapist within individual teams to organize "team huddles" at the beginning of each workday. These discussions could also be scheduled in a routine that is appropriate for each particular work environment. The purpose of these huddles is to briefly discuss each client's therapeutic status and treatment requirements, including clients who are needing both occupational therapy and physiotherapy. These team discussions will assist the OTAs and PTAs in planning their daily work schedules; this results in more effective and positive client outcomes by providing the therapy treatments required by each client on a timely basis.

References

Association of Canadian Occupational Therapy Regulatory Organizations, Association of Canadian Occupational Therapy University Programs, & Canadian Association of Occupational Therapists. (2021). *Competencies for occupational therapists in Canada.* OT-Competency-Document-EN-HiRes.pdf (acotro-acore.org)

Association of Canadian Occupational Therapy Regulatory Organizations (ACOTRO). (2019). *ACOTRO Position statement regarding utilizing occupational therapist assistants in occupational therapy service delivery.* https://acotro-acore.org/wp-content/uploads/2021/10/20190226_acotro_position_statement_-_ota_and_regulation_of_ot_-_revised_final_revised.pdf

Bellefontaine, K., Hurley, M., & Irngaut, S. (2015). Community therapy assistant: Supporting rehabilitation services in the remote arctic community of Igloolik, Nunavut. *Occupational Therapy Now, 17*(2), 21–22.

Blake, M., Park, D., & Brice-Leddy, L. (2015). Occupational therapists as practice managers, assistants as primary providers of therapeutic interventions: It's time to talk. *Occupational Therapy Now, 17*(2), 13–15.

Caines, A. (2015). Use of an occupational therapist assistant in food exposure intervention for preschoolers with autism spectrum disorder. *Occupational Therapy Now, 17*(2), 6–7.

Canadian Association of Occupational Therapists. (2024). *Competencies for occupational therapist assistants.* https://caot.ca/document/8146/Competencies%20OTA%20EN%20Feb%208%202024.pdf

Canadian Association of Occupational Therapists. (2022–23). *Professional Liability Insurance brochure.* https://caot.ca/document/5794/CAOT_PLI_Brochure.pdf

Canadian Physiotherapy Association. (2023–24). *PTA Professional Liability Insurance brochure.* https://physiotherapy.ca/app/uploads/2024/03/CPA_PTA_Brochure_2023-2024.pdf

College of Occupational Therapists of British Columbia. (2023). *Practice standard for supervision of occupational therapist assistants.* https://cotbc.org/library/cotbc-standards/practice-standards-and-guidelines/

Gerber, S. (2022). *Emotional magnetism: How to communicate to ignite connection in your relationships.* Vancouver: NEXT IMPACT Press.

Gillespie, H. (2023). Occupational therapist and OTA collaboration: The how is now. *Occupational Therapy Now, 26*(6), 9–12.

Hagler, P., Madill, H., & Kennedy, L. (1994). Facing choices about our beliefs regarding support personnel. *Canadian Journal of Occupational Therapy, 61*(4), 215–218.

Newfoundland and Labrador Occupational Therapy Board. (2021). *Practice guideline: Task assignment to assistants in occupational therapy service delivery.* https://www.nlotb.ca/images/pdf/2021/legislation_and_guiding_documents/Practice-Guideline-Task-Assignment-to-Assistants-NLOTB-January-2020.pdf

World Federation of Occupational Therapists. (2024). *Guiding principles for ethical occupational therapy.* https://wfot.org/resources/wfot-guiding-principles-for-ethical-occupational-therapy

4

Evaluating Occupational Therapy Service Delivery

Objectives

After completing this chapter, the reader will be able to:

♦ Describe potential methods to evaluate client outcomes through occupational therapist and OTA collaboration.
♦ Reflect on OTA involvement on improving clients' well-being.
♦ Understand how to more consistently improve clients' occupational participation through collaboration with OTAs.
♦ Recognize that collaborating with OTAs provides occupational therapists with increased opportunities to complete additional work requirements.
♦ Apply the benefits of the collaboration to timely and effective healthcare delivery.

Key Terms

♦ Intraprofessional collaboration evaluation
♦ Potential self-evaluation tools

DOI: 10.4324/9781003498391-4

- Client satisfaction and well-being
- Occupational participation
- Further recommended research

Frequently Asked Questions (FAQs) are included at the end of this chapter.

Evaluation Processes

It is important for the supervising occupational therapist to ensure that the OTA (or OTAs) to whom they have assigned client treatments provide consistent, safe, and timely therapies, and that the outcome results in optimal client and/or caregiver satisfaction. This is an area that requires further research in order to provide concrete evidence of positive outcomes resulting from involvement of OTAs in the delivery of occupational therapy treatments.

As described in Chapter 3, it is necessary for the supervising therapist to clearly understand the OTA role as well as the competence of each OTA to whom they potentially assign activities to facilitate the client's occupational participation. One method the occupational therapist can use to achieve this understanding is through reviewing and evaluating the OTA's work with each client, particularly if the therapist and the OTA are entering a new therapeutic working relationship. It is also necessary to reflect on the results of the collaboration between the therapist and the OTA throughout the performance of the assigned activities.

A potential evaluation process to determine the degree of effective client outcomes through collaboration between the occupational therapist, the OTA, and the client will be described. Although the completion of this type of evaluation will increase the workload for the occupational therapist to a certain extent, it will assist the therapist in determining whether changes need to be made within their assignment and supervision practices. The frequency of completing this type of evaluation would depend on the occupational therapist's experiences working with specific OTAs and the overall workplace policies.

The initial part of this evaluation process is a client satisfaction questionnaire administered by the supervising occupational therapist who had assigned the client treatments to the OTA(s). If more than one OTA was included within the assignment to this client, the therapist must ensure that all OTAs are referred to within the questions.

The questions asked of the client could include:

1. Do you recall the OTA(s) who provided you recent treatment? (*Identify the specific treatments being referred to*)
2. Did they arrive as scheduled for each visit and stay for the planned length of time?
3. Was the treatment's purpose and process explained to you prior to beginning the session?
4. Were you asked to provide consent preceding the treatment being initiated?
5. Did the OTA(s) consider your cultural safety?
6. Were you comfortable to ask the OTA(s) any questions during the treatment?
7. If so, did the OTA(s) answer your questions clearly?
8. Do you agree that the treatment provided was successful in reaching the following goals we agreed to following my initial occupational therapy assessment with you? The goals I am referring to include:
   Goal #1
   Goal #2
   Goal #3
9. Would you agree to receive treatments by the OTA(s) in the future?
10. Overall, how would you rate this occupational therapy experience on a scale from 1 to 10, with 1 being unacceptable and 10 being excellent?

The results of this subjective questionnaire will provide detailed information about the assigning of these specific treatments to the OTA (or OTAs) which the supervising occupational therapist can examine, and may contribute to changes that may need to be made in the future. The strategies to incorporate these changes could include further training for the OTA related to this treatment or providing education about alternate ways to approach the client in explaining the treatment. It also could positively reinforce that the competencies the OTA demonstrated while treating this client are evidence of the OTA's skills and knowledge, indicating the appropriateness of assigning this task in future clinical situations.

In addition to the subjective information received, the supervising occupational therapist will gather objective data by completing a reassessment of the client. This reassessment will provide evidence as to changes within the client's abilities as well as any continuing limitations following delivery of the treatment by the OTA(s). This would assist in answering the following questions:

- ◆ Have the client's objectives and goals been met?
- ◆ Has the treatment provided by the OTA improved the client's overall well-being?

A further component to this evaluation could include a review of the workload requirements that the supervising occupational therapist was able to complete while the OTA(s) were delivering treatments to the client. This collaboration between the therapist and the OTA will result in more time available for the therapist to meet other obligations within their job description as the OTA(s) are providing the treatments. Examples of responsibilities the occupational therapist would have more time to complete could include:

- ◆ Completing "X" number of client initial assessments, reassessments, or potential discharge assessments.
- ◆ Initiating and/or completing required documentation requesting third-party funding for assistive devices and/or equipment required by a client in order to remain living safely at home.

◆ Participating in required discussions with medical vendors to solve specific issues related to a client's equipment needs.

◆ Providing direction to teachers and staff within the school system regarding procedures to incorporate in the classroom for students with specific needs.

◆ Educating executives and employees as to involving occupational therapy for those with specific needs to access occupational participation within their facility or organization. This could include service areas within the justice system, driver rehabilitation programs, and childcare centres, as well as recommending universal design to community officials to promote accessibility within local public buildings.

◆ Initiating communications with local contractors to discuss becoming involved in home renovations for clients wanting to age in place.

◆ Attending an interprofessional team meeting to discuss a client's situation with family members.

◆ Mentoring a new occupational therapist colleague on developing effective therapeutic collaborative relationships with the OTAs within their work environment.

This is a potential method of evaluating the benefits in assigning tasks to the OTA(s) in all work settings for both the clients' positive outcomes as well as effective and timely healthcare delivery. In addition, evidence would support that occupational therapists can make additional time available to complete further professional responsibilities when collaborating more consistently with OTAs in the provision of client treatments.

Outcomes from the Occupational Therapist and OTA Collaboration

This section will discuss positive outcomes that have resulted from occupational therapists and OTAs working together in a trusting and effective working relationship. These examples are within a Canadian context and are based on research studies or observations and reflections from rehabilitation managers and staff.

1. **Therapist assistants supporting improved patient flow in a hospital setting**

   Blandford discusses the benefits of involving occupational therapists in managing patient flow through interprofessional collaboration and including therapist assistants in treatment delivery. The setting is a general hospital environment and the clients involved had experienced a brain injury or cerebrovascular accident (CVA). An occupational therapist and a speech language pathologist collaborated with home care teams, including assigning rehabilitation treatments to therapist assistants, to "create a home-based rehabilitation plan for selected clients and navigate them home early by providing their final week of therapy in the client's home" (Blandford, 2018, p. 29). Based on this change in service delivery involving assistants, a "total of 509 bed days were saved in a 12-month period" (Blandford, 2018, p. 29).

2. **Enhancement of the OTA/PTA role within a teaching hospital**

   Blake, Park, and Brice-Leddy review an innovative practice change that was initiated within a large teaching hospital. OTAs and PTAs became primary providers of therapy interventions, and the occupational therapists and physiotherapists became practice managers and were mainly involved in patient assessment, treatment planning, and discharge planning (Blake, Park, & Brice-Leddy, 2015, p. 13). Occupational therapy interventions were provided mainly by OTAs seven days a week and baseline competencies were established to cover rotation on various units within the hospital. This also applied to physiotherapy interventions, but occupational therapy will be the main focus in this context. Occupational therapists needed to ensure that each OTA was competent in the clinical skills required on each particular unit and provided training when needed. Time was also taken to ensure that all team members understood the OTA role and that occupational therapists continued to maintain responsibility for occupational therapy interventions. During a review of the project, "participants felt strongly that patients were being seen more frequently and benefiting from the enhanced services of OTA/PTAs" (Blake, Park, & Brice-Leddy, 2015, p. 14).

A qualitative study later reviewed how this new model of care in acute medicine affected therapists' practice and patient outcomes. Semi-structured interviews were conducted with four occupational therapists and four physiotherapists. The general result was that "overall, they thought that the enhanced availability of care provided by OTA/PTAs was beneficial to patients because they received more frequent and consistent care" (Brice-Leddy, Park, Bateman, Drysdale, Ratushny, Musse, & Nixon, 2020, p. 174). However, the therapists also described "difficulties of transitioning from being a provider of patient care to a manager of patient care provided by assistants" (Brice-Leddy, Park, Bateman, Drysdale, Ratushny, Musse, & Nixon, 2020, p. 174). Recommendations from this study include the following:

♦ Enhanced communication, trust, and accountability between occupational therapists, physiotherapists, and OTA/PTAs need to be developed.
♦ Effective supervision skills need to be taught to therapists in their formal education program.
♦ Increased time available for therapists to interact with assistants to exchange information and to ensure OTA/PTAs are performing competently.
♦ Opportunities for continuous learning for OTA/PTAs.
♦ Occupational therapy and physiotherapy professions to incorporate the competencies required to supervise multiple assistants within their competency frameworks.

(Brice-Leddy, Park, Bateman, Drysdale, Ratushny, Musse, & Nixon, 2020)

Of note, the final recommendation from this study aligns within Domain A, *Occupational Therapy Expertise*, from the 2021 *Competencies for Occupational Therapists in Canada*:

The competent occupational therapist is expected to

◆ **A7 Manage the assignment of services to assistants and others**
  • **A7.1** Identify practice situations where clients may benefit from services assigned to assistants or others.
  • **A7.2** Assign services only to assistants and others who are competent to deliver the services.
  • **A7.3** Monitor the safety and effectiveness of assignments through supervision, mentoring, teaching, and coaching.
  • **A7.4** Follow the regulatory guidance for assigning and supervising services.
      (ACOTRO, ACOTUP, CAOT, 2021, p. 11)

3. **OTAs teaching clients to practice operating power mobility devices**
  Gillespie and Engel discuss OTAs becoming involved in a power mobility training program within a community where the older population is experiencing increasing challenges with mobility and limitations in driving motor vehicles (Gillespie & Engel, 2015, p. 8). OTA positions were created within the home care program due to increasing caseload demands within occupational therapy, and one treatment that was regularly assigned to OTAs was power mobility training. The occupational therapist would decide whether to assign this training to the OTA based on the risks involved and, if assigned, the therapist would then document the requirements of the training within the supervision plan. The occupational therapist would ensure that the OTA and the specific medical vendor who provided the mobility device for the practice trial would develop an effective working

relationship for scheduling and planning purposes. The OTA would document in the health record following each practice session and the occupational therapist would review the documentation to determine any graded alterations that needed to be incorporated within the assignment (Gillespie & Engel, 2015, p. 9). This process was regularly reviewed, and numerous clients achieved safe driving skills while operating the power wheelchair or power scooter and expressed confidence in their abilities. The advantages of including the OTA in power mobility training are as follows:

1. "Although the occupational therapist is responsible for the intervention, the OTA in this program has developed skills and knowledge required for power mobility training through experiences with other occupational therapists and clients within the home care program. The OTA has become vital to the learning experience of current clients" (Gillespie & Engel, 2015, p. 9).

2. The OTA can "provide individualized suggestions to the client, such as those related to route choices, navigation through certain areas such as parking lots, and access to public transit" (Gillespie & Engel, 2015, p. 9).

3. Clients receive "individualized attention that would not be available in the occupational therapist's schedule and caseload" (Gillespie & Engel, 2015, p. 9).

The success of this program emphasizes the benefits of a collaborative working relationship and effective communication between the supervising occupational therapist and the OTA to improve clients' occupational participation and quality of life.

A further example of the importance in building this collaboration to benefit a client's power mobility training is based on the author's experience while working in a community setting. The OTA had been assigned power wheelchair training for a client living within the city environment. The client needed to cross one busy road to access public services, but the OTA reported to the author that the client could not activate the pedestrian crossing lights at the crosswalk due to a decorative gravel base surrounding the pole that contained the crosswalk button. The gravel base prevented the client from moving the power wheelchair close enough for them to reach the button. The author contacted the city engineering department to report this concern regarding the infrastructure and was informed that it would be investigated. When the OTA returned to this same crosswalk the following day with the client, the gravel base had been removed and the client was able to push the button allowing traffic to stop and was then able to safely cross the street. The communication between the OTA and the occupational therapist initiated this opportunity to improve community access for this client, and likely many others who rely on power mobility devices within the area.

4. **Increasing the role of OTAs within a hospital setting**
   Vo and Feenstra review the development of their OTA role within an urban teaching hospital by collecting data on OTAs' responsibilities from various acute care units over a six-month period (Vo & Feenstra, 2015, p. 23). The statistics demonstrated that a considerable amount of time was spent on wheelchair seating interventions which included providing an appropriate wheelchair for each client, completing adjustments and modifications as required, and educating the client in using the seatbelt and brakes correctly and in how to mobilize the wheelchair safely. Although this is an appropriate role for OTAs, there are many more benefits that the OTAs could provide within a hospital environment. This resulted in the development of a *Reference Guide to the Roles of an OTA* document which was shared with the occupational therapists within the workplace. In addition, an Assistant Education Committee was created that "organized eleven educational sessions over three years for assistants working in various acute care areas" (Vo and Feenstra, 2015, p. 23). The result of these initiatives was increased involvement of OTAs in direct patient treatments other

than wheelchair seating, which "enabled the occupational therapists to focus more on new consults and discharge planning" (Vo & Feenstra, 2015, p. 23).

The initiatives taken by OTAs within this setting gave rise to an expanded OTA role in delivering patient treatments which provided the occupational therapists with more time to complete their responsibilities in a more timely manner, resulting in overall improved patient care.

Frequently Asked Questions

1. **How can we provide evidence to demonstrate the positive outcomes that residents experience from occupational therapist and OTA collaborations within long-term care facilities?**

   Occupational therapy provided within long-term care facilities is an area where increased research studies need to be completed within Canada to objectively demonstrate the positive outcomes achieved for residents when OTAs are involved with therapy delivery. This action has been strongly encouraged across the country for an extended period of time.

   General observations can be made and documented by occupational therapists and OTAs based on certain therapy treatments within current facilities which could include the following:

   ◆ Residents have demonstrated an increase in independence in certain activities following treatments provided by the OTA such as being able to feed themselves using adapted utensils.

   ◆ There are fewer issues with skin integrity for residents required to rely on a wheelchair for seating and mobility challenges. This has been more evident since the occupational therapist and OTA have collaborated to obtain the most appropriate size and style of wheelchair for each resident along with the required cushion and supports. The OTA monitors the wheelchair fit regularly and checks on the correct use and inflation of the cushion as needed.

◆ The residents who had previously required regular behavior modification medication due to increased anxiety are needing this medication less frequently as their anxiety levels have decreased. This has occurred since the OTA initiated leisure activities that are enjoyed by residents, with craft projects, singing groups, and playing board games as a few examples. The OTA has developed a trusting relationship with each resident and with their family members if possible, and has learned about special interests or hobbies the resident previously participated in. The OTA has taken this additional knowledge and applied it to specific activities for the individual resident.

◆ Certain residents are requiring less pain medication since they have participated in exercise classes directed by the OTA. They can work within their abilities and the exercises are graded as necessary. The results of this additional strengthening have improved mobility and general functioning beyond what was evident prior to the exercise class being available.

◆ With agreement and confirmation from the facility manager, the occupational therapist was able to connect with the manager of a local child daycare organization. It was agreed that staff from the daycare would bring a group of children to the long-term care facility on a regular schedule and the children along with certain residents in the care facility would work together on a project that was facilitated by the OTA. The activities could include coloring a picture together, putting together an easy jigsaw puzzle, or playing a simple board game. The OTA could also organize smaller groups where a resident could read a story to a few children and encourage engagement in conversation between the resident and the children about the story.

The author experienced a similar situation in a care home where children were brought to the facility once a week. One resident was hesitant to participate in other occupations but regularly joined the children in activities when they visited the facility. The positive outcome for this resident was evident in their facial expression, body language, and engagement with the children.

2. **If OTAs are involved in treating injured workers, is there evidence that the workers can recover sooner and return to work earlier than if OTAs were not involved?** The author is not aware of specific research that has been completed in Canada on this topic, but OTAs are frequently involved in rehabilitation programs for workers who have been injured on the job. Funding for the involvement of OTAs would have to be approved from the worker's compensation funder prior to involving the OTAs in treatment. Based on the successful evidence of OTAs within other treatment settings resulting in positive client outcomes, as reviewed in previous chapters, it is likely that similar results would occur with this client population. The OTAs would need to demonstrate competence on the required work simulation activities to enable specific clients to be able to return to their job. If this was a new activity for the OTA, they would need to receive appropriate training as needed. If it was required that the OTA visit a specific job site for further client treatment or observation, and this was approved by the workplace, funder, and the supervising therapist along with the client, this would further ensure that the most appropriate treatment was being provided to the client and would likely expedite their return to work.

As frequently discussed throughout the book, the client would be able to receive more timely and efficient occupational therapy if an OTA was assigned specific treatments to perform, rather than this being an additional responsibility for the supervising occupational therapist. This would allow the therapist to assess more clients, and complete the required documentation and funding requests on a timelier basis; the client would also benefit by likely being able to return to work in a more opportune time frame.

References

Association of Canadian Occupational Therapy Regulatory Organizations, Association of Canadian Occupational Therapy University Programs, & Canadian Association of Occupational Therapists. (2021). *Competencies for occupational therapists in Canada*. OT-Competency-Document-EN-HiRes.pdf (acotro-acore.org)

Blake, M., Park, D., & Brice-Leddy, L. (2015). Occupational therapists as practice managers, assistants as primary providers of therapeutic interventions: It's time to talk. *Occupational Therapy Now, 17*(2), 13–15.

Blandford, M. (2018). Occupational therapists and patient flow: Important contributions and opportunities to make a difference. *Occupational Therapy Now, 20*(4), 27–29.

Brice-Leddy, L., Park, D., Bateman, W., Drysdale, J., Ratushny, L., Musse, S. & Nixon, S.A. (2020). Enabling access to rehabilitation in acute care: Exploring physiotherapists' and occupational therapists' perspectives on patient care when assistants become the primary therapy providers. *Physiotherapy Canada, 72*(2), 169–176. doi.org/10.3138/ptc-2018-0073

Gillespie, H. & Engel, L. (2015). Occupational therapist assistants: Enabling well-being in community power mobility users. *Occupational Therapy Now, 17*(2), 8–10.

Vo, L. & Feenstra, C. (2015). The emerging role of occupational therapist assistants at the Ottawa Hospital. *Occupational Therapy Now, 17*(2), 23.

5

Future Growth of Occupational Therapy with an Evolving OTA Role

Objectives

After completing this chapter, the reader will be able to:

♦ Encourage further learning by student occupational therapists as to the OTA role.
♦ Describe the benefits of the occupational therapist and OTA collaboration.
♦ Support OTA professional development education opportunities.
♦ Increase managers' understanding of the OTA role.
♦ Learn potential OTA involvement of in additional practice settings.
♦ Utilize a self-evaluation tool for OTAs to complete in collaboration with supervising occupational therapists.

Key Terms

♦ Intraprofessional student collaboration
♦ Employment requirements for OTAs

DOI: 10.4324/9781003498391-5

- ◆ Improvement of therapist and team clarity of the OTA role
- ◆ Professional development
- ◆ Role-emerging OTA practice areas
- ◆ Mentoring
- ◆ Self-evaluation
- ◆ OTA and PTA Vision Project

Frequently Asked Questions (FAQs) are included at the end of this chapter.

Future Student Collaboration

Chapter 1 discussed the success of intraprofessional student collaboration within fieldwork placements where student occupational therapists and OTA students learn together from the same occupational therapist preceptor, including learning about each other's roles and responsibilities. There were also situations discussed where therapist and OTA students worked on projects together within their education programs or learned certain practical skills within a healthcare environment. Discussions with occupational therapist professors have indicated that OTAs have recently been hired within occupational therapist master's education programs at various universities across the country to provide education to the student occupational therapists. It is understood that the OTAs in these positions teach the student therapists about their roles within client treatments and their responsibilities in reporting to the supervising occupational therapists. Although this is not a true "intraprofessional student collaboration" example as only student occupational therapists are involved, it does ensure that student therapists are learning about the role of their intraprofessional colleagues to whom they will be assigning client treatments within their career.

The author experienced an intraprofessional student collaboration while employed in the manager role within a hospital therapy department. The idea of offering an intraprofessional fieldwork experience was deliberated within the rehabilitation team, resulting in a physiotherapist agreeing to be the preceptor for both a physiotherapist student and a PTA student. This opportunity was organized through discussions with the university physiotherapist education program and the therapist assistant education program within the same province. The results of the placement experience for all involved were positive, although it did create extra work for the physiotherapist preceptor. However, it was agreed that the positive experiences of both students as to learning about each other's roles outweighed the additional required responsibilities.

This experience corroborates with the literature studies discussed in Chapter 1 which found that intraprofessional placements are critical to both student therapists and student therapist assistants learning about each other's responsibilities within specific clinical settings. It is strongly encouraged that these combined fieldwork placement experiences are organized more consistently across the country to benefit student occupational therapists and OTA students as they begin their careers. Understanding that fieldwork placements vary in length and are scheduled differently within each program, discussions still need to take place to potentially offer some flexibility in the scheduling which could result in this collaboration occurring more regularly. This is reiterated by Stephenson who states, "Educators of occupational therapy, physical therapy and therapist assistant programs are encouraged to explore intraprofessional education opportunities. Problem-based learning sessions and joint fieldwork placement experiences are avenues for exploring roles and responsibilities, task assignment, supervision, effective communication and the value of intraprofessional relationship building" (Stephenson, 2015, p. 28).

As discussed in Chapter 1, along with these education opportunities occurring within occupational therapy, Francis and Strader said that they "encourage others to establish interprofessional education or IPE units in hospitals across Canada. Increased opportunities and support for IPE across the country would enable OTA and PTA education programs to provide their students with the foundational knowledge and skills necessary to demonstrate optimal interprofessional competence" (Francis and Strader, 2015, p. 30).

To summarize this topic, education programs for student occupational therapists and OTA students need to have a more consistent collaboration to incorporate intraprofessional and interprofessional learning opportunities within their training. The outcome of this recommendation is that students will graduate having a stronger understanding of the importance of collaboration within their upcoming occupational therapy careers.

A presentation by Francis at the 2017 CAOT Conference on the results of a study in 2015 titled *OTA & PTA Graduates' Transitions into Clinical Practice* indicated that therapist assistants graduating from a two-year accredited diploma program demonstrated the following capabilities:

1. Problem-solve and think critically
2. Prioritize tasks
3. Promote safety during patient/client interactions and
4. Carry out treatment plans assigned by the occupational therapist and physiotherapist.

This study demonstrates an understanding and confidence by OTA and PTA graduates in their role and that they are competent to make valuable contributions to therapy services (Francis, CAOT Conference, 2017). This brings up the same question that is frequently asked: If therapist assistants who graduate from an accredited education program are able to demonstrate competencies in skills they have learned, why are they not more involved in the therapy team? As repeatedly discussed in previous chapters, the response to this question is often related to the lack of understanding as to their role by others within healthcare, and this needs to improve in the near future. Although it is questionable whether accreditation of OTA and PTA education programs should become mandatory, the education standard these students receive from an accredited program would provide a baseline for therapists and employers to better understand the abilities and knowledge of therapist assistants. This increased role clarity can then be applied to building and supporting therapist and assistant working relationships and can also be incorporated during the provision of client treatments.

Improve the Occupational Therapist and OTA Collaboration

The mixed-methods study by Penner and colleagues in 2020, *Viewpoints of the Occupational Therapist Assistant – Physiotherapist Assistant Role on Interprofessional Teams*, discusses five emerging themes on the therapist/assistant collaboration, some of which were highlighted in Chapter 2. In summary, these themes are listed below:

1. **Left out of the loop**: Assistants voiced concerns about communication, inclusion, and opportunities for continuing education compared with their therapist colleagues – and this has been reiterated by other assistants across the country. "The assistants felt marginalized when they were not given a choice to participate by being either directly or indirectly excluded from educational opportunities" (Penner, Snively, Packham, Henderson, Principi, & Malstrom, 2020, p. 399). This theme also applies to the assistants not being included within team and family meetings, or being asked to provide updates within rounds even though they spend most of their time treating clients (Penner, Snively, Packham, Henderson, Principi, & Malstrom, 2020).

2. **Living in the grey – negotiating and navigating the OTA/PTA role**: what actually is the role of therapist assistants? The challenge is that their role is very broad and is greatly determined by the relationship that is developed between the therapists and the assistants. Their role can also be confusing as they are dual trained and may work with clients providing one area of therapy, possibly physiotherapy which then results in a lack of skill development within the other profession, in this case occupational therapy (Penner, Snively, Packham, Henderson, Principi, & Malstrom, 2020).

3. **Who's the boss**? Issues of power and power structures affect daily practice. Therapist assistants feel conflicting accountability between supervising therapists and managers resulting from the "therapists' lack of training as supervisors, unclear or conflicting accountability to therapist supervisors versus unit managers, and disempowering or devaluing hierarchies" (Penner, Snively, Packham, Henderson, Principi, & Malstrom, 2020, p. 401).

4. **Things don't just fall in your lap – pursuing professional development**: Assistants identified a lack of continuing education opportunities and a lack of funding support including paid time to attend a course or workshop. Additionally, assistants feel marginalized when courses specify a health degree as a prerequisite (Penner, Snively, Packham, Henderson, Principi, & Malstrom, 2020).

5. **(Not) just an assistant – the influence of norms and attitudes and external perspectives**: OTAs and PTAs need to assert that they are "not just assistants but core team members who make valuable contributions to team function and client care" (Penner, Snively, Packham, Henderson, Principi, & Malstrom, 2020, p. 402). Another observation within this study was that therapists often referred to assistants as "my assistant." This description should not be used as it can imply "dominance intended to reinforce hierarchy and power differentials" (Penner, Snively, Packham, Henderson, Principi, & Malstrom, 2020, p. 402).

The occupational therapist and OTA collaboration needs to be better understood and refined as a means of improving access to, and cost-effectiveness of, occupational therapy service delivery. A potential means through which this could be achieved within the provinces where occupational therapists are regulated could be that therapists need to complete an online learning module as a registration requirement, which could be updated annually as required. To ensure consistency, the module would need to be based on the practice standard or guideline for assigning and supervising OTAs within the regulatory college. The learning from this module would be one way to increase their confidence and competence in assigning tasks and supervising OTAs.

Continuous professional development activities and courses are needed to update professionals' knowledge and skills within their work setting. This definitely applies to occupational therapists and OTAs who should be able to attend professional development workshops or courses either as a team or individually, based on their learning needs. This learning could focus on new client treatments, assistive devices, or equipment in addition to other resources related to occupational therapy. An example experienced by the author was attending an education session on new mobility devices available to local clients. The OTA working with the author in the community work setting also attended. During the medical vendor's description about a new mobility device, and which types of clients it could benefit, the OTA turned to the author and stated, "this device would be a great option for client X." The author agreed with the OTA and, following a successful practice trial assigned by the author and completed by the OTA with the medical vendor, this new device was funded for the client.

OTAs also need to complete courses that will increase their skillset and the types of client populations they are confident to treat. This type of professional development may result in a specialized certification within a certain practice area which could increase the OTA's job opportunities or update their understanding of providing new treatments to a specific client population.

The ongoing learning for OTAs throughout their career aligns with Domain D, *Excellence in Practice*, within the *2024 Competencies for Occupational Therapist Assistants*, which states:

The competent OTA is expected to:

◆ **D1 Engage in ongoing learning and professional development**
  - **D1.1** Develop professional development plans.
  - **D1.2** Demonstrate awareness of required competence to meet job requirements.

- **D1.3** Determine resources to enhance knowledge, skills, behaviour, and attitudes.
- **D1.4** Engage in professional development activities to improve practice and ensure continuing competence.

(CAOT, 2024, p. 10)

It is common knowledge that professional development courses can be costly to complete and often require a short-term leave from the workplace. OTAs need to be able to receive funding assistance to participate in new learning opportunities in addition to being allowed a paid leave of absence. It is understood that current workload pressures can make this challenging in certain work environments, but enabling the OTAs to increase their knowledge and skills will increase the occupational therapy services that can be provided within the workplace. An additional current concern when attempting to register for certain courses is the requirement for the registrant to have a specific education credential that is often not necessary for professional development. This type of requirement needs to be removed for courses that can be completed by OTAs with various educational backgrounds with the result of increased competencies and benefit to the clients.

Employers and managers also need to invest time in learning more about the role of therapist assistants, the occupational therapist and OTA relationship, and the importance of therapist assistants on the interprofessional teams. This information can be learned through reviewing resources from professional occupational therapy associations, regulatory colleges, and OTA education programs. Another means of achieving this education is by attending an in-person or virtual workshop on topics related to the occupational therapist and OTA collaboration. In addition, OTAs need to be encouraged to educate the leaders, managers, and employers within their workplace as to their general role within occupational therapy for specific client populations as well as sharing their individual competency skills. OTA/PTAs can also explain how they can work in both occupational therapy and physiotherapy while following the supervision requirements for each profession.

Chapter 3 references a new model of therapy delivery within an acute care hospital where OTAs became the primary providers of therapeutic interventions. To ensure therapist and assistant collaboration, Blake, Park, and Brice-Leddy describe a learning needs assessment that was developed for the OTA/PTAs to confirm that they could demonstrate the competencies needed to treat the clients. This was followed by the initiation of a clinical learning environment to assist the assistants in learning those skills they lacked in order to increase the supervising therapists' confidence in assigning these tasks to all OTA/PTAs on each hospital unit (Blake, Park, and Brice-Leddy, 2015, p. 13).

The management team needs to be open and supportive to learning which will assist in supporting the rehabilitation team to provide optimal care for those in need. This is reinforced by Stephenson, "For optimal engagement of the assistant by therapists, department or program managers and organizations, there must be an understanding of the assistant's education, scope of practice, roles and responsibilities. Opportunities for team building activities should be considered to promote intraprofessional and collaborative team development. Collegial learning opportunities, such as joint program planning and encouraging the therapist and assistant to attend continuing education sessions together, can promote discussions regarding the application of content to intraprofessional practice" (Stephenson, 2015, p. 28). Supporting OTAs in their continuing education through attendance at workshops or providing updated resources on practice updates will ultimately result in expanding the occupational therapy practice within the clinical environment.

This aligns with the final competency within Domain D, *Excellence in Practice*, within the *2024 Competencies for Occupational Therapist Assistants*, which states:

The competent OTA is expected to:

◆ **D3 Monitor developments in practice**
  - **D3.1** Stay aware of political, social, economic, environmental, and technological effects on occupational therapy practice.

- **D3.2** Keep up to date with research guidelines, protocols, and practices.
- **D3.3** Integrate relevant evidence into practice.

(CAOT, 2024, p. 10)

Increase OTA Involvement in Selected Occupational Therapy Treatments

A few occupational therapy treatments involving OTAs are described below to demonstrate certain clinical practice areas and work settings that could increase collaboration between occupational therapists and OTAs in the future.

1. Caines describes developing food acceptance for children with autism spectrum disorder (ASD) as "a long-term process requiring regular exposure sessions as well as parental involvement" (Caines, 2015, p. 6). One-on-one sessions are often more successful, particularly for clients who are less socially motivated. This can include "demonstrating how to play with food at the table, identifying different levels of food acceptance, demonstrating positive interactions with a variety of different foods and showing how to integrate other approaches into a session, such as positive reinforcement, behavioural modification and total communication" (Caines, 2015, p. 6). The occupational therapist is not able to provide the frequency of visits the client requires due to workload, resulting in the assignment of these treatments to a competent OTA who can provide the client and their parents with a consistent approach. The OTA documents observations following each session with the client, and these are reviewed by the occupational therapist.

   The OTA who is involved in this clinical setting has received specific training on sensory feeding approaches and techniques in addition to desensitization and play-based learning. The OTA is also an active member of the food exposure committee within the work setting (Caines, 2015, p. 7).

The OTA is supervised either directly or indirectly by the occupational therapist depending on the situation, and they collaborate to problem-solve together as issues arise. Any questions asked by the parents to the OTA are forwarded to the supervising occupational therapist who addresses their questions (Caines, 2015).

"Having the OTA help provide food exposure is crucial to success of the intervention as there is not enough time for the occupational therapist to work in depth on the food issues the client may have" (Caines, 2015, p. 7).

2. Increased OTA involvement within long-term care facilities has been previously discussed in this book. The number of people in such facilities is continuing to grow due to the increased lifespan experienced in Canada, and because many of the older citizens are unable to live alone in their own homes as they require a certain amount of assistance with home maintenance and/or personal care. The inclusion of occupational therapy within long-term care facilities is critical as a means to maintain or improve each resident's quality of life through participation in meaningful occupations for as long as possible. Occupational therapists can be hired or contracted on a part-time basis for two or three days a week and OTAs are often hired or contracted full-time. The OTAs can work under the remote supervision of the occupational therapists on days when the therapists are not working at the facility and follow the documented supervision and communication plan for each resident. In this type of healthcare environment, the OTAs will develop strong therapeutic relationships with the residents as they treat them on a regular basis over a long period of time. The OTAs will also be able to collaborate with the supervising occupational therapists when certain needs change for a resident, requiring a re-assessment and development of a new treatment plan by the occupational therapist.

This team approach will result in positive outcomes for everyone involved.

3. Certain children within the school system would greatly benefit from an increase in occupational therapy treatments to improve their learning and concentration abilities. These therapies can be provided by an OTA under the supervision of an occupational therapist. Examples of these treatments could be:

- A child with autism spectrum disorder (ASD) may benefit from wearing a weighted vest to calm them when they have sensory processing issues as the vest helps with sensory regulation. The OTA can ensure the proper fit of the weighted vest for the child and follow up by educating the teacher, EA, and the parents on the wearing requirements.

- Another option for increasing the focus for children with ASD could be to use noise-cancelling headphones, and the OTA can be assigned to assist the child in learning when and how to apply the headphones and to educate the teacher and the child's parents in the correct use of these headphones.

- A student with cerebral palsy requires the use of a specialized wheelchair. The OTA can review the proper fit of the wheelchair, and adjust it as required for the student to successfully perform activities at their desk in the classroom. The OTA can educate the teacher on the requirements needed for a correct fit and demonstrate how to make the adjustments if required. If the wheelchair is powered, the OTA can also instruct the school staff on how the wheelchair operates and on the most effective method and schedule of charging the battery when needed.

- A child with fine motor issues can be taught to use a large pencil or an adapted writing device to improve their focus on handwriting. This could result in an increased ability to focus on written tasks within their classroom. The OTA could monitor that the child is using the pencil correctly and instruct the teacher on the correct use of the pencil.

- A teen with obsessive compulsive disorder (OCD) may require exposure and response prevention (ERP) therapy to be able to focus better within their classroom. This therapy could be provided by an OTA who has received specific training in the delivery of ERP, and who would report to the supervising occupational therapist as documented in the supervision plan.

4. As well as staff shortages and limited resources within certain hospital environments, concerns are raised about wait times for some services including rehabilitation. The involvement of more OTAs in addition to PTAs within all hospital areas will increase the therapy services that are available to those needing this care. Although positive examples are demonstrated in many facilities, as described previously in this book, the involvement of competent OTAs should continually increase in order to provide the necessary occupational therapy services. Managers of both therapists and OTAs within rehabilitation programs need to encourage increased safe and appropriate assignment of therapy treatments more consistently.

Related to this last statement, it is critical that therapists are included within the decision-making process when therapist assistants are being hired, as the occupational therapists and physiotherapists will be working with the OTA/PTAs and are accountable for their client interventions and safety. This was included in the mixed-methods study by Penner and colleagues in 2020 within *Theme 3: Who's the boss?*. A concern expressed by therapist participants was that they were "excluded from hiring and staffing decisions about assistants or other support personnel under their supervision as 'That's the managers' decision'" (Penner, Snively, Packham, Henderson, Principi, & Malstrom, 2020, p. 401).

OTAs Orientating Occupational Therapists and Students to Their Role

This topic aligns with Domain F, *Engagement Within Occupational Therapy*, within the *2024 Competencies for Occupational Therapist Assistants*, which states:

> **The competent OTA is expected to:**
>
> ◆ **F1 Contribute to the learning of occupational therapists, OTAs, and others**
> - **F1.1** Contribute to entry-to-practice education, such as fieldwork placements.
> - **F1.2** Facilitate continuing professional development activities.
> - **F1.3** Act as a mentor or coach.
> ◆ **F2 Show leadership in the workplace**
> - **F2.1** Support OTAs, student OTAs, student occupational therapists, and other colleagues and team members as appropriate.
> - **F2.2** Influence colleagues to progress toward workplace values, vision, and goals.
> - **F2.3** Support improvement initiatives at work.
> - **F2.4** Serve as a role model.
> - **F2.5** Act responsibly when there are environmental or social impacts to their own behavior and consult with the supervising occupational therapist as needed.
>
> (CAOT, 2024, p. 12)

Some of these indicators are demonstrated by Vo and Fenestra, as discussed in Chapter 4, which addresses the development of their *Reference Guide to the Roles of an OTA* document which was shared with the occupational therapists within the workplace and the Assistant Education Committee that was created to provide ongoing education for OTAs (Vo and Feenstra, 2015, p. 23). This was also discussed by Debra Cooper in her dialogue within Chapter 2, saying that OTAs need to be involved in educating and mentoring others as to their skills and to act as a role model. This includes educating student occupational therapists within their university coursework and during fieldwork placements, initiating education sessions with staff occupational therapists who have never collaborated previously with OTAs, and being encouraged to educate leaders and managers who are unaware of their role and responsibilities as OTAs. This could be more defined, with OTAs being members or chairs of continuing education committees within healthcare organizations to allow them to provide input into education sessions or workshops that are required for the staff from an OTA perspective.

Role-Emerging OTA Practice Areas

Expanding the role of OTAs within role-emerging areas of practice aligns with Domain F, *Engagement within Occupational Therapy*, within the 2024 CAOT *Competencies for Occupational Therapist Assistants*:

> **The competent OTA is expected to:**
>
> ◆ **F4 Show leadership in occupational therapy throughout career**
>   - **F4.1** Promote the value of OTAs within occupation and occupational therapy in the wider community.
>   - **F4.2** Advocate for the involvement of OTAs within occupational therapy standards and processes, organizational policies, social justice, and emerging best practices.
>   - **F4.3** Take part in occupational therapy and community activities, such as volunteering for events and committees.
>   - **F4.4** Influence the profession and its contribution to society.
>
> (CAOT, 2024, p. 12)

Examples of opportunities to further incorporate this competency and indicators will be further discussed.

Chapter 1 of this book briefly suggested expansion of the occupational therapy profession in various areas. This included role-emerging fieldwork placements for both student occupational therapists and OTA students – and potentially experiencing this type of fieldwork together. Another area that has evolved due to the recent pandemic is virtual healthcare delivery that has involved many medical professions including occupational therapy. This is a way that therapists can remotely supervise assistants providing therapy when each is in a different geographical location. An example of this type of remote supervision, as discussed by Bellefontaine, Hurley, and Irngaut, was included in Chapter 3. Although this type of collaboration can be more challenging when safe and operative communication technology is required, it does provide those residing in remote locations with the opportunity to access the therapy services they require on a timely basis (Bellefontaine, Hurley, and Irngaut, 2015, p. 22).

Promoting wellness and injury prevention is becoming more prevalent in current healthcare systems. OTAs need to be more involved in providing this type of education to recipients in a variety of programs which would enable a range of learning resources to be more accessible to an increased number of individuals and families.

The opportunity to grow occupational therapy service delivery across the country is continuing to evolve, and it is necessary to increase the collaboration of the occupational therapist and OTA team to achieve the optimal outcome for everyone involved. The role of OTAs within certain locations is advancing to include additional work environments, client populations, and treatments. New practice areas can be established through the advocacy of occupational therapists, educators, and team leaders in various practice areas who understand the OTA role and the therapist regulatory requirements for assigning and supervising, and recognize the need for increased occupational therapy involvement across the country.

Examples and brief descriptions of role-emerging OTA practice areas and increased involvement within current practice areas are described below.

- ◆ A population that could benefit from increased involvement of the occupational therapist/OTA team is those with mental health conditions. Practice settings could include homeless shelters, community mental health centres, and mental health facilities. An example of this type of setting was shared by an occupational therapist colleague. This particular treatment site includes a mental health program that provides art classes for those in the community and is run by OTAs who are supervised by an occupational therapist. This setting provides a safe environment that is supportive and enables healing, and many of the volunteers who assist with the program are former group members.

- ◆ OTAs can be assigned to educate seniors who are interested in aging in place. Following a home assessment by the occupational therapist, the OTA can follow up by suggesting certain processes and devices that are commonly recommended for fall and injury prevention. These can include, but are not limited to, the following:
  - Suggesting that seniors de-clutter their home environment a couple of times a year.
  - Placing a chair at the front door or garage door so that they can sit down while putting on and taking off their shoes.
  - Recommending that stairs are well lit and have safe railings on both sides that are regularly maintained, and that there is non-slip tread on the steps. Another option that could be discussed for future use is a stair glide which would be beneficial if the homeowners begin to experience mobility issues. If they asked the OTA about whom to contact for any of these home modifications, the OTA would inform the occupational therapist, who would then follow up with the clients.

- Strongly encouraging the use of non-slip mats within their shower stall or bathtub as well as on the floor outside the shower unit. Grab bars also need to be installed, if possible, to improve safe access into and out of the tub or shower. The OTA would reinforce that soap dish handles or curtain rods are not to be used in place of grab bars. A consideration for the homeowners is to potentially renovate the bathroom by installing a wheel-in shower with no threshold or a built-in seat, and this could be further discussed with the occupational therapist.
- Increasing the height of the toilet by using a raised toilet seat or replacing the current toilet with one that is higher. This assists with easier transfers on and off based on the user's height.
- If they enjoy gardening, installing raised planting beds can make this occupation easier to enjoy for a longer period of time.
- If they need to use a walking device such as a cane or walker but are hesitant to do so due to the stigma surrounding their use, the OTA can reinforce that these devices are no different than using a TV remote device or a garage door opening device – they simply make life easier.

◆ CarFit is an occupational therapy educational program for drivers to improve their comfort behind the wheel while driving their vehicle. The program was created by the American Occupational Therapy Association along with the American Automobile Association and AARP. Within Canada, CarFit is jointly supported by CAOT and the Canadian Automobile Association (CAA) (CAOT, 2024). CarFIt focuses mainly on educating older drivers as to their best fit within their vehicle, resulting in a safer driving experience. CarFit events are organized and hosted by a Carfit coordinator who has previously been trained as a CarFit technician.

CarFit technician training is free to complete and those that can apply for the training include Canadian registered or retired occupational therapists, student occupational therapists, and OTAs. The training requires completing an online or in-person classroom session in addition to an in-person CarFit event. The in-person training could also be completed virtually if required. Following their training, the role of the occupational therapy practitioner is educating drivers who attend the CarFit events, and is described on the CAOT website (CarFit - CAOT). Components of this education process completed by the technicians include reviewing the following:

- Position of the driver's seat in relation to the steering wheel
- Seat belt is worn correctly
- Steering wheel properly tilted
- Distance between the chest and airbag
- Line of sight above the steering wheel
- If a head restraint is in place, it is properly adjusted
- The gas and brake pedals can be fully depressed (and clutch if applicable)
- Proper mirror position
- Operation of vehicle controls
- Awareness of vehicle technologies
- Final review and checkout

(CAOT & CAA, 2024)

It is clearly stated in the CarFit Occupational Therapy Practitioner Role document on the CAOT website that "At no time does the OT practitioner provide individual occupational therapy interventions. The role is to provide education only, it is not intended to be therapy or therapeutic intervention" (CAOT, 2024, p. 1).

OTAs are strongly encouraged to become involved in the CarFit program. Although being a CarFit practitioner is a volunteer position, OTAs in addition to occupational therapists and student occupational therapists play an extremely important role in educating the older population in the occupation of driving. The drivers are provided with the required information and resources they can utilize to assist with their safety while driving.

◆ OTAs are becoming more involved in wheelchair seating clinics within healthcare settings. They have learned through their education programs how to determine the best wheelchair fit for individual clients and how to adjust them as needed when the client's status changes. Knowledge about the added supports, cushions, and adaptations that are available are also within their skillset, and OTAs are often the most appropriate staff members to be responsible for maintaining wheelchairs that are loaned to clients within hospital and long-term care settings until it is determined by the occupational therapist that a permanent wheelchair is required.

◆ Within certain practice settings, OTAs work with clients to assist them in accessing public buildings. This may involve recommending an easier entrance that the client could use, teaching them how to access a device that assists in opening doors, the safest method to access elevators, or how to utilize a ramp. Throughout this experience, the OTAs learn about specific challenges the clients may experience in certain public spaces and can often provide options for improvements to the supervising occupational therapist. Together the therapist and the OTA can advocate for improved universal design to promote accessibility within local public buildings. Examples of these recommendations could include adding railings to stairways, installing grab bars beside toilets in public washrooms, providing easy to read and clear directions to direct users to services within the building, adding ramps to entrances, improving lighting at the entrance and throughout buildings, or widening doorways for easier wheelchair access.

◆ Online education for those who want to pursue a career as an occupational therapist or OTA, or for an OTA who wants to advance their education to become an occupational therapist, provides access for those living in remote communities as well as individuals who are unable to attend in-person programs due to personal and/or family reasons. There are currently OTA education programs that are provided online and this opportunity could continue to increase. In addition, there is a need to create accessible online occupational therapy master's education programs for those who are unable to relocate to attend an in-person program. As referenced in Chapter 1 from the recently published *Joint Position Statement – Toward Equity and Justice: Enacting an Intersectional Approach to Social Accountability in Occupational Therapy*, there is the recommendation within the Education section: "Create accessible occupational therapy programs with varied delivery options to meet diverse access needs (e.g. part-time, online and weekend programs, virtual and in-person fieldwork placements), that can be delivered with and in underserved communities" (CAOT, ACOTRO, ACOTUP, 2024, p. 11).

OTA and PTA Vision Project

The occupational therapist assistant (OTA) and physiotherapist assistant (PTA) Vision Project (Vision OTA PTA) was initiated in 2017. The project's purpose was to discuss the future of OTAs and PTAs within Canada and it brought together various stakeholders to participate in the dialogues. As stated in the Executive Summary, "Despite the ongoing evolution of OTA/PTA practice in Canada, there is no single organization/body which represents the OTA/PTA perspective, nor an agreed-upon vision of how these important healthcare team members can best contribute to the health and wellness of Canadians in partnership with occupational and physiotherapists" (ACOTRO, ACOTUP, CAOT, CAPR, CCPUP, COPEC, CPA, OTA & PTA EAP, PEAC, 2019, p. 1). Stakeholders came together initially in Stage 1 through a national survey in 2017 which identified specific areas that required more discussion. This was followed by Stage 2, which involved two phases of focus group discussions in 2018 that further explored these key areas (ACOTRO, ACOTUP, CAOT, CAPR, CCPUP, COPEC, CPA, OTA & PTA EAP, PEAC,

2019, p. 1). The Executive Summary 2019 describes the qualitative and iterative methodology used in Stage 2 and includes key messages and recommendations that are presented not in order of priority but in order of the online discussions. Examples are:

◆ **Recommend creation and better communication of educational materials to support standards of practice for supervision of OTA/PTAs**

It was acknowledged that one of the challenges with assigning tasks to OTA/PTAs is the limitation of time provided to occupational therapists and physiotherapists s for supervision requirements in addition to the variability of the competencies of practicing OTA/PTAs. It is also stated that many occupational therapists and physiotherapists do not recognize OTA/PTA competencies that can be safely delivered during treatment delivery. On the contrary, occupational therapists and physiotherapists may not be aware of their own regulatory supervision requirements and assign tasks beyond the competence of the OTA/PTA.

As OTA/PTAs need to work to their full potential within the supervising therapists' regulations, it is necessary that occupational therapists and physiotherapists be aware of regulatory standards regarding assignment and supervision within their province, and the OTA/PTAs must also be aware of their own limitations. This reinforces that therapists must apply their regulated practice standards or guidelines when collaborating with OTA/PTAs.

(ACOTRO, ACOTUP, CAOT, CAPR, CCPUP, COPEC, CPA, OTA & PTA EAP, PEAC, 2019, pp. 2–3)

◆ **Recommend investigating the feasibility of a certification program through CAOT/CPA**

Discussions on the development of a registry, a national certification program, and/or regulation for OTA/PTAs occurred during the focus groups. It was generally agreed that inclusion on a registry which incorporated the use of a consistent title coupled with standards and a certification process would be valuable. This could "assist in standardization if employers were to adopt the practice of hiring only those certified by a national association" (ACOTRO, ACOTUP, CAOT, CAPR, CCPUP, COPEC, CPA, OTA & PTA EAP, PEAC, 2019, p. 3). The participants understood that certification would not ensure protection of title. It is interesting to note that from the focus groups, approximately 70% of OTA/PTAs supported regulation and employers, educators, and regulators generally did not support regulation.

> (ACOTRO, ACOTUP, CAOT, CAPR, CCPUP, COPEC, CPA, OTA & PTA EAP, PEAC, 2019, p. 3)

◆ **Recommend exploring the creation of a joint CAOT/ CPA membership tier for OTA/PTAs**
General support of a Collaborative Joint Group within the Canadian Association of Occupational Therapists (CAOT) and the Canadian Physiotherapy Association (CPA) was favoured rather than OTAs and PTAs forming their own national association. The joint collaboration would better align with the dual education of OTA/PTAs, would facilitate higher membership numbers, and would better support certification and/or registration.

> (ACOTRO, ACOTUP, CAOT, CAPR, CCPUP, COPEC, CPA, OTA & PTA EAP, PEAC, 2019, p. 4)

◆ **Recommend use of consistent title**
It was strongly recommended by 95% that a consistent title nationally be used. The preference within the group was slightly in favour of the title Occupational Therapist Assistant/Physiotherapist Assistant to be used in contexts where assistants are working under

the supervision of an occupational therapist and/or physiotherapist. The term "therapist" within the title was preferred over "therapy" as it provides further clarity to everyone involved in the therapy delivery that the OTA/PTAs are "assisting" the occupational therapist and/or physiotherapist in their delivery of the therapy treatment.

(ACOTRO, ACOTUP, CAOT, CAPR, CCPUP,
COPEC, CPA, OTA & PTA EAP,
PEAC, 2019, pp. 4–5)

The title of Therapist Assistant is also strongly recommended based on the confusion that can occur when the designations of "support personnel" or "rehabilitation assistant" are used in organizations. These titles give a poor understanding of the roles of the assistants and their responsibilities to team members as well as to clients and family members. This lack of clarity can also place the supervising therapists in challenging ethical situations when they are asked to assign to assistants who may not have the competencies required to perform the specific treatment needed by the client.

◆ **Recommend creation of a dual competency profile**
  Currently, there are separate OTA and PTA competency profiles. Participants were provided with the following description of a dual profile:
  A dual profile would include competencies common to both OTAs and PTAs that are required of both disciplines (e.g., ethics, professionalism, communication, record keeping). At the technical skill level, the profile would diverge and include OTA-specific and PTA-specific skill-level competencies. Assistants practising in only one discipline would be held to the common competencies and the skill-level competencies of the one discipline. Thus, the profile would be applicable to single trained/practising OTAs, single trained/practising PTAs and to dual trained/practising OTA/PTAs.
  (ACOTRO, ACOTUP, CAOT, CAPR, CCPUP, COPEC,
  CPA, OTA & PTA EAP, PEAC, 2019, p. 5)

It was generally agreed that a development of a dual competency profile would better align competencies with education programs/accreditation and the practice environment. A dual competency would also play a role in potential certification in the future.

As of the writing of this book, no updates on the Vision Project recommendations are available.

OTAs' Self-Evaluation within Occupational Therapy Treatments

The new OTA competencies have provided the occupational therapy team with a resource that clarifies the OTA role and incorporates updated occupational therapy terminology. Descriptions of culture, equity, and justice are also clearly expressed in order to increase inclusion and understanding. The term "competencies" within the document refers to skills that can be demonstrated and they reflect a broad range of OTA skills and abilities. The competencies required in various situations will be influenced by and depend on the model of care and/or the client (individuals, groups, communities, or populations), where the work is being done, and the needs of the client. Individual OTA competence in a specific treatment must be determined by the occupational therapist based on these factors prior to assigning the treatment (CAOT, 2024, p. 2).

As discussed in Chapter 4, assessing the client outcomes following occupational therapy treatment is required to determine the next steps including adjustments to the treatment plan based on the client's progression or regression in meeting their goals, initiating a new treatment plan to meet a new target, discharging the client if they have met their goals, or discontinuing treatment if the client is no longer consenting to or capable of continuing with therapy.

It is also beneficial for healthcare providers to complete regular self-evaluations to determine if they are meeting the competencies and standards as a regulated healthcare professional within their specific healthcare environment. Although OTAs are not regulated within Canada, it would be beneficial to the intra-professional and interprofessional teams for each OTA to evaluate their performance within their work setting in collaboration with their supervising occupational therapists. The results of these self-evaluations can then provide recommendations and objectives for potential professional development education, required updates to team processes, and review of the collaborative therapist/assistant relationship including effective communication. In addition, this evaluation process could validate each OTA's contribution to occupational therapy treatment delivery and possibly expand their role as appropriate within the work environment.

An example of a self-evaluation tool was developed by the author based on the 2024 CAOT *Competencies for Occupational Therapist Assistants*. This evaluation has not been utilized to date, but the concept could be incorporated as an assessment tool to enable work settings to review the contribution of OTAs to the profession of occupational therapy. The evaluation is provided below:

OTAs' Self-Reflection Tool in Collaboration with Supervising Occupational Therapists:

Name _____

Date_____

Supervising Occupational Therapist_____

1. I understand my role and responsibilities and share this with clients and team members as required.
    0) Disagree   1) Somewhat Agree   2) Agree   3) Strongly Agree   Comments:

2. I work within the ethics, rules and regulations that govern occupational therapy within my work environment.
    0) Disagree   1) Somewhat Agree   2) Agree   3) Strongly Agree   Comments:

3. I promote equity and cultural safety within my practice.

0) Disagree   1) Somewhat Agree   2) Agree   3) Strongly Agree   Comments:

4. Client safety and minimizing risk is of optimal importance within my clinical practice.

0) Disagree   1) Somewhat Agree   2) Agree   3) Strongly Agree   Comments:

5. I communicate with my supervisor(s) as required in the documented supervision plan for each client.

0) Disagree   1) Somewhat Agree   2) Agree   3) Strongly Agree   Comments:

6. I am comfortable approaching my supervising therapist(s).

0) Disagree   1) Somewhat Agree   2) Agree   3) Strongly Agree   Comments:

7. I incorporate problem-solving and critical thinking into my practice as required and collaborate with the supervising occupational therapist(s) as needed.

0) Disagree   1) Somewhat Agree   2) Agree   3) Strongly Agree   Comments:

8. I maintain documentation following each client treatment that meets the organization's requirements.

0) Disagree   1) Somewhat Agree   2) Agree   3) Strongly Agree   Comments:

9. I have participated in professional development activities and review available educational resources as needed to meet my professional development plan.

0) Disagree   1) Somewhat Agree   2) Agree   3) Strongly Agree   Comments:

10. I contribute to the growth of occupational therapy through supporting colleagues, student occupational therapists, and OTA students.

0) Disagree   1) Somewhat Agree   2) Agree

3) Strongly Agree   Comments:

This type of self-reflection tool aligns with Domain D, Excellence in Practice, within the 2024 CAOT *Competencies for Occupational Therapist Assistants*:

The competent OTA is expected to:
- ◆ **D2 Improve practice through self-assessment and reflection**
  - **D2.1** Self-evaluate using performance and quality indicators.
  - **D2.2** Learn from varied sources of information and feedback.
  - **D2.3** Contribute to the process of giving feedback to others when required.
  - **D2.4** Manage work resources and demands effectively.
  - **D2.5** Be mindful of occupational balance and wellbeing.

(CAOT, 2024, p. 10)

Frequently Asked Questions

1. **Why has the word "assess" not been used more when a component of an OTA's role is "assessing" a client's progress to determine how the treatment they are providing is progressing?**

   This is a question that often arises and can be very confusing for both therapists and OTAs. It does need to be clear in the communication if a specific occupational therapy assessment tool is involved as these are often completed by an occupational therapist "especially if clinical judgment is required" (ACOTRO, 2019, p. 1). If the term "assess" is related to an OTA commenting that "when I assessed client J's ability to complete the hand exercises this afternoon compared to our session three days ago, the required repetitions of each exercise were achieved today," this can be an acceptable use of the word "assess." Differentiating between "assessment" that a therapist completes and "assessment" that an OTA completes has at times been made by using "Assessment" for a therapist and "assessment" for an OTA. Other comparisons of this terminology may be that a therapist "evaluates" a client's abilities, and an assistant "assesses" the client's progress during treatment.

Based on this confusion, the author does recommend that this terminology be clarified in the future to ensure it is clear to everyone if an OTA can "assess" a client's progress through incorporating the critical thinking skills they have learned in their education, or if another term should be used, such as "monitoring" or "observing". However, the latter two terms may result in a decrease in the critical thinking used by the OTA during client treatment sessions.

2. **Is it being considered that accreditation of OTA and PTA education programs may become mandatory?**
   This question has been raised in workshops and conferences, and there have been differing opinions and issues regarding the establishment of this requirement in the future. Education programs that are not currently accredited have expressed concerns particularly related to the amount of work involved to prepare for accreditation and the cost of the process to their institutions. The positive consequence of mandatory education accreditation is that therapists, managers, and employers would understand the foundational knowledge and skills of the OTA/PTAs they hire as each one would have needed to meet the accreditation standards required for graduation. As has been discussed frequently throughout this book, there currently is a lack of understanding of particularly the OTA role by key stakeholders involved in occupational

therapy, and mandatory accreditation would assist in improving this knowledge.

Another option for consideration resulted from the Vision OTA PTA project discussed earlier in this chapter and it involves initiating a certification process for OTA/PTAs. This could "assist in standardization if employers adopt the practice of hiring only those certified by a national association" and "would ensure that those OTA/PTAs who are not graduates of an accredited education program have a way to demonstrate they meet the same standard of care" (ACOTRO, ACOTUP, CAOT, CAPR, CCPUP, COPEC, CPA, OTA & PTA EAP, PEAC, 2019, p. 3).

References

Association of Canadian Occupational Therapy Regulatory Organizations (ACOTRO), Association of Canadian Occupational Therapy University Programs (ACOTUP), Canadian Association of Occupational Therapy (CAOT), Canadian Alliance of Physiotherapy Regulators (CAPR), Canadian Council of Physiotherapy University Programs (CCPUP), Canadian Occupational Therapist Assistant & Physiotherapist Assistant Educators Council (COPEC), Canadian Physiotherapy Association (CPA), Occupational Therapist Assistant & Physiotherapist Assistant Education Accreditation Program (OTA & PTA EAP), Physiotherapy Education Accreditation Canada (PEAC). 2019. *Vision OTA PTA executive summary*. Vision OTA PTA (caot.ca)

Association of Canadian Occupational Therapy Regulatory Organizations. (2019). *ACOTRO position statement regarding utilizing occupational therapist assistants in occupational therapy service delivery*. https://acotro-acore.org/wp-content/uploads/2021/10/20190226_acotro_position_statement_-_ota_and_regulation_of_ot_-_revised_final_revised.pdf

Bellefontaine, K., Hurley, M., & Irngaut, S. (2015). Community therapy assistant: Supporting rehabilitation services in the remote arctic community of Igloolik, Nunavut. *Occupational Therapy Now, 17*(2), 21–22.

Blake, M., Park, D., & Brice-Leddy, L. (2015). Occupational therapists as practice managers, assistants as primary providers of therapeutic interventions: It's time to talk. *Occupational Therapy Now, 17*(2), 13–15.

Caines, A. (2015). Use of an occupational therapist assistant in food exposure intervention for preschoolers with autism spectrum disorder. *Occupational Therapy Now, 17*(2), 6–7.

Canadian Association of Occupational Therapists. (2024). *Competencies for occupational therapist assistants.* https://caot.ca/document/8146/Competencies%20OTA%20EN%20Feb%208%202024.pdf

Canadian Association of Occupational Therapists, Association of Canadian Occupational Therapy Regulatory Organizations, & Association of Canadian Occupational Therapy University Programs. (2024). *Joint position statement – Toward equity and justice: Enacting an intersectional approach to social accountability in occupational therapy.* https://caot.ca/document/8179/Toward%20Equity%20and%20Justice_JPS_EN_V3.pdf

Canadian Association of Occupational Therapists and Canadian Automobile Association (COAT). (2024). *CarFit.* CarFit - CAOT.

Canadian Association of Occupational Therapists and Canadian Automobile Association. (2024). *Carfit: Occupational Therapy Practitioner Role.* CarFit Occupational Therapy Practitioner Role.pdf (caot.ca)

Francis, D. (2017). *Transitioning into clinical practice: Occupational therapist and physiotherapist assistant graduates perceptions of clinical competence. CAOT Conference Presentation.* Charlottetown, PEI.

Francis, D. and Strader, C. (2015). The role of occupational therapist assistant and physiotherapist assistant students on an interprofessional education unit. *Occupational Therapy Now, 17*(2), 29–30.

Penner, J., Snively, A., Packham, T., Henderson, J., Principi, E., & Malstrom, B. (2020). Viewpoints of the occupational therapist assistant – Physiotherapist assistant role on inter-professional teams: A mixed-methods study. *Physiotherapy Canada, 72*(4), 394–405. https://doi.org/10.3138/ptc-2019-0011

Stephenson, J. (2015). Working together: Today's dynamic duo! *Occupational Therapy Now, 17*(2), 28.

Vo, L. & Feenstra, C. (2015). The emerging role of occupational therapist assistants at the Ottawa Hospital. *Occupational Therapy Now, 17*(2), 23.

Conclusion

The content within this book has discussed the information on the occupational therapist and OTA collaboration that is needed to be understood and applied within the occupational therapy profession. Although the education of OTAs is variable across Canada, the voluntary education accreditation program provides a standardized knowledge and skill level for graduates from these programs. The benefits of both intraprofessional and interprofessional components within education programs can improve these collaborations when entering the workforce by increasing awareness of each team member's roles including those of occupational therapists and the OTAs. Cultural safety needs to be a requirement within occupational therapy education on a more consistent level to improve students' understanding of incorporating culture, equity, and justice within their upcoming career.

The initial process in creating a successful occupational therapist and OTA team is by developing a trusting professional relationship. Processes that can assist in forming this relationship are discussed from the author's career experience and through the perspective of an OTA. It is also imperative that managers, practice leaders, and employers within all health care systems support these processes as well as allowing the time that is required for this successful collaboration to develop. Learning to effectively communicate is critical within any relationship and a procedure has been described within the book to assist in accomplishing this requirement. The topic of ethics is reviewed, including a decision-making process to approach ethical dilemmas within occupational therapy. Examples from the author's perspective provide possible solutions to these situations.

Understanding the treatment assignment process that an occupational therapist utilizes when involving an OTA in therapy can

DOI: 10.4324/9781003498391-6

be difficult to apply within various clinical situations. Although certain specific requirements may differ within provincial regulatory organizations, a general decision to assign procedure is included along with case examples. Once the occupational therapist decides to assign a treatment to OTAs, a supervision and communication plan is documented, and the author has included examples to provide further clarification. Documentation by OTAs is discussed although this will vary within all practice areas and organizations. The topic of professional liability insurance is also reviewed.

Evaluating the outcomes resulting from OTAs improving clients' occupational participation needs to be completed on a more regular basis across the country. This includes initiating research studies across occupational therapy practice areas. Potential processes for this type of evaluation have been included, in addition to literature reviews within Canada.

The future growth of OTAs within occupational therapy is discussed in Chapter 5. This includes increasing intraprofessional student collaboration, clarifying the OTA role to healthcare teams, promoting professional development education for OTAs to encourage ongoing learning, and developing potential role-emerging practice areas within occupational therapy.

In summary, OTAs are extremely valuable members of the occupational therapy profession and need to receive more recognition and support for their contributions. Increased successful occupational therapist and OTA collaborations will result in timely and cost-effective occupational therapy treatments to improve the occupational participation and overall quality of life of Canadians.

Index

Printed in the United States
by Baker & Taylor Publisher Services